THE GERM HANDBOOK

LESLIE ANN DAUPHIN, PhD

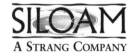

A STRANG COMPANY

Most STRANG COMMUNICATIONS/CHARISMA HOUSE/SILOAM products are available at special quantity discounts for bulk purchase for sales promotions, premiums, fund-raising, and educational needs. For details, write Strang Communications/ Charisma House/Siloam, 600 Rinehart Road, Lake Mary, Florida 32746, or telephone (407) 333-0600.

THE GERM HANDBOOK by Leslie Ann Dauphin, PhD
Published by Siloam
A Strang Company
600 Rinehart Road
Lake Mary, Florida 32746
www.siloam.com

Unless otherwise noted, all Scripture quotations are from the King James Version of the Bible.

Scripture quotations marked AMP are from the Amplified Bible. Old Testament copyright © 1965, 1987 by the Zondervan Corporation. The Amplified New Testament copyright © 1954, 1958, 1987 by the Lockman Foundation. Used by permission.

Cover design by Judith McKittrick
Interior design by Terry Clifton

Library of Congress Cataloging-in-Publication Data
Dauphin, Leslie Ann.
  The germ handbook / Leslie Ann Dauphin.
    p. cm.
  Includes bibliographical references.
  ISBN 1-59185-786-4 (pbk.)
  1. Medicine, Popular. 2. Communicable diseases. 3. Medical microbiology. 4. Health--Religious aspects--Christianity. I. Title.
  RC81.D2297 2005
  616.9'0471--dc22
                    2005005392

Author's note: This book is an independent endeavor by the author, and it is not endorsed by the CDC.

People and incidents in this book are composites created by the author. Any similarity between the names and stories of individuals described in this book to individuals known to readers is purely coincidental.

Neither the publisher nor the author is engaged in rendering professional advice or services to the individual reader. The ideas, procedures, and suggestions in this book are not intended as a substitute for consulting with your physician. All matters regarding your health require medical supervision. Neither the author nor the publisher shall be liable or responsible for any loss or damage allegedly arising from any information or suggestion in this book.

05 06 07 08 — 987654321
Printed in the United States of America

DEDICATION

To my two fathers: my biological father, Charles Williams, who is the best any daughter could hope for, and my spiritual father, Dr. Creflo Dollar. They have provided spiritual covering, guidance, and instruction. They inspire me, and I thank God for them both.

CONTENTS

INTRODUCTION

Gary has not done well in school this year. In fact, his grades have been awful. His teacher suggests that he may have to repeat the third grade if there is no improvement. Excessive absences have affected his performance in school. Gary's mother argues that his absences are due to illnesses that could not be controlled and are excused. She makes the case that on two different occasions Gary had the "sniffles," but she sent him to school anyway, and he was sent home. As with many schools in the United States, the policy at Jackson Elementary School requires that sick students stay home. If a student is present and there is any indication of a contagious illness (fever, runny nose), the parent is called and the student is sent home. Gary's teacher feels sympathetic, but the truth is that Gary is unable to keep up with the rest of the class and will probably be held back.

Of course, this story is an extreme case of what can happen as a result of sickness leading to poor attendance at school. However, many students in schools across the country do not perform to the best of their ability because of excessive illness-related absences. In a survey conducted by the Centers for Disease Control and Prevention's (CDC) National Center for Health Statistics, it was found that of the country's 53 million school-aged children, 6 percent (3.2 million) missed more than 11 days of school due to illness or injury.[1] Illnesses such as colds, flu, and other respiratory diseases caused by germs have a great impact on both children and adults. Among the country's 119,000 schools, the flu has caused high rates of absenteeism among students and staff.[2] The CDC reports that an estimated 22 million school days each year are lost due to the common cold alone.[3]

Just imagine how many parents are absent from work to nurse their sick children back to health. That number is probably high as well. Maybe you have been one of them! The good news is that Gary and his parents can have better control over his health. It is reported that students miss fewer days of school when they practice healthy habits.

THE ENEMY

As a youngster I was very interested in the human body, but I was never interested in becoming a medical doctor. I always knew that treating sick people was an awesome call, but not the call for *my* life. Instead, I was drawn to learn about preventing sicknesses and diseases. This led to the study of microbiology, the science of small (*micro*) living things (*biology*) or germs. I wanted to understand the things that made people sick and to learn of ways to prevent the diseases they cause. Since completing my doctorate degree and while working at the CDC, I have gained knowledge about the simple practices that prevent the spread of infectious diseases. One of the reasons I have written this book is to share basic practices that can be applied to people's lives to help prevent many of the diseases caused by germs.

In this book I refer to the germs that cause diseases in our bodies as "the enemy," because in many ways they operate as the enemy does. The Bible states that the thief comes not but to steal, to kill, and to destroy (John 10:10). That is exactly what these germs do to our bodies. Germs *take space* in our bodies without obtaining our permission (steal). When we are infected by them, they often cause damage to our bodies and affect our well-being (destroy). Many of the diseases caused by them can lead to death (kill), especially in unhealthy or elderly people. When we are stricken with an infectious illness, we are unhappy and unproductive. We are far less capable of working to carry out God's purpose for our lives.

KNOWLEDGE AS A DEFENSE

We've all heard the phrase "knowledge is power." So in order to better defend ourselves against the enemy (germs), we need to know the enemy and know how it will attack us. Armed with the correct information, we can apply many simple practices in our daily lives to defend ourselves against the enemy.

It's easy to feel overwhelmed by the technical information issued by the health department. Too often people rely on the media to "decode" this jargon for them, which can lead to misinformation. One goal of this book is to teach, in simple terms, about the germs that are responsible for some of the common illnesses that we encounter. If you learn what these germs are and how they spread to cause infection, then you will be better prepared to defend yourself against them and the diseases that they can bring to your life.

> For wisdom is a defense even as money is a defense,
> but the excellency of knowledge is that wisdom
> shields and preserves the life of him who has it.
> —ECCLESIASTES 7:12, AMP

By reading this book you will learn:

- The four types of germs that cause infectious diseases
- How germs are spread and make us sick
- The germs that receive attention from the media
- Myths vs. truth about common infectious diseases
- Myths vs. truth about immunizations
- What vaccines are, how they work, and the types of vaccines used today
- The types of treatments used for infectious diseases
- The side effects associated with treatments for infectious diseases
- Common infections we can get from our pets
- The link between germs and chronic diseases such as cancer, heart disease, and arthritis
- Scientific and biblical practices to prevent common infectious diseases
- How to take care of your body to maintain health
- The power of prayer and a good attitude for maintaining health

Many people believe that science and the Bible are conflicting. Nothing could be further from the truth. This belief is due in part to a misunderstanding of science and the Bible. It has become clear to me that much of what we are currently learning in the sciences has already been outlined in the Bible. Actually, in many ways, science is just beginning to catch up with the information in the Bible. The preventive measures currently advised by the CDC are plainly written throughout the Bible: seeking knowledge and wisdom (education), practicing cleanliness, having healthy eating habits (avoiding gluttony), taking care of the body (cleansing the temple), and avoiding unsafe behaviors are just some of the many examples.

POWER FROM GOD AS A DEFENSE

Part of the defense strategy against germs is knowing how to apply biblical principles in your daily life to keep yourself and loved ones from sickness and disease. This is not a book about healing, but rather one about germs and how to keep them from getting you sick. The Bible tells us to seek wisdom. (See Proverbs 4.) In doing so, we become aware of things that we can do to prevent sickness and disease from occurring. Applying the knowledge you gain from this book will help you defend yourself against the enemy in the natural, while applying the knowledge of God's Word will help you defend against the enemy in the spiritual sense. What the sciences are missing is an understanding of God's power. Those who have God in their lives, however, can receive His power, which is the ultimate defense against the enemy.

> Behold, I give unto you power to tread on serpents
> and scorpions, and over all the power of the enemy:
> and nothing shall by any means hurt you.
> —Luke 10:19

Many of the natural preventive measures advised by health scientists are already described in the Bible and are, therefore, "spiritual."

Another goal of this book is to compare preventive measures described by health professionals versus those described in the Bible, which is why you will read many Scripture references in this book. I encourage you, therefore, to spend time reading, meditating, and applying these scriptures to your life daily.

UNIT 1

THE ENEMY

Chapter 1

GERMS: WHAT THEY ARE

Germs. They are everywhere. Most of these organisms are not harmful, but if your immune system is weak, it can leave you vulnerable to infectious diseases. The issue is that the public knows very little about what germs are and how they operate. If you are going to defeat the enemy, you first need to know the enemy.

In order to help you understand how germs attack your body, let me take you back to your grade school science class. Try to remember what it was like growing "stuff" in a little dish and learning about viruses, bacteria, cells, and the like. In this chapter I will cover four basic types of infectious agents: viruses, bacteria, parasites, and fungi. They are characterized by their types of cells, the basic unit of life. All contain representatives that may be infectious and may cause a range of infections from very mild to fatal.

VIRUSES (THE USERS)

Imagine how you would feel if someone came into your home without permission and took control of everything you own. My guess is that you would feel awful. You would probably want to do whatever is necessary to get rid of the home invader and prevent him from ever entering your home again.

This is what viruses do to our bodies—invade, take control, and make us feel awful. Viruses lack the basic units of life—cells—so they invade our bodies because they are unable to survive on their own. While everything that is living is made up of cells, viruses are simply made up of genetic material (*genome*) and protein (Fig. 1). They use *our* cells to carry out *their* life functions. For example, viruses cannot reproduce on their own. They use the materials in our cells to make copies of themselves. Imagine that! Our cells serve as surrogates. Viruses are indeed *users* of our bodies.

Viruses are grouped based on their structure and are also referred to by the name of the disease they cause. For example, the virus that causes AIDS is a retrovirus (genus) and is referred to as the human immunodeficiency virus or the AIDS virus (disease). Viruses are much smaller than bacteria. So small, in fact, that they require a special, high-powered microscope to view them with our eyes. According to the American Society for Microbiology, viruses can be as much as 10,000 times smaller than bacteria.[1] Examples of common diseases in humans caused by viruses are colds, flu, and chickenpox.

Of all the germs to study, I find viruses the most interesting. They are responsible for so many of the diseases for which there is no cure, and they are the most puzzling. Many of the infections that lead to lifelong disability are caused by viruses. These include AIDS, polio, and shingles. They are capable of infecting all forms of life, including plants, animals, and even other germs. Viruses are the most diverse of all the germs on earth.

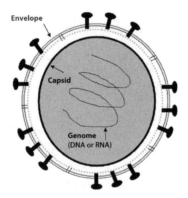

FIGURE 1. Above is a cartoon representation of the basic structure of a virus. Viruses are composed of genetic material (genome) and a protein coat called capsid. Some viruses contain an outer layer called an envelope, which may contain other structural proteins.

BACTERIA (THE NUISANCES)

Many people understand more about bacteria and preventing bacterial infections than they probably think. For example, what is the first thing a person does when they get a cut or scrape? They quickly use something to clean the wound and then cover it with a bandage. They know that if they don't, it can become infected. What about the mother preparing a chicken dinner for her family? She carefully washes her hands, cleans surfaces in the kitchen, and rinses the chicken before cooking. She believes that this may prevent her family from getting sick. These actions indicate an understanding of the most important fact about bacteria: they are everywhere. Unlike viruses, bacteria are made up of cells and are therefore capable of survival on their own. And, boy, do they do a great job of it! They survive in the foods we eat, the water we drink, and even on us. The truth is, it is impossible to get away from them, which is why they can be somewhat of a nuisance.

BACTERIAL SHAPES[2]

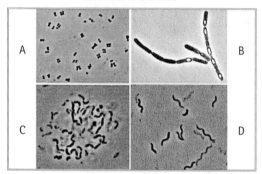

FIGURE 2. Above are micrographs of bacteria representing four basic shapes: spherical (cocci), rod shaped (bacilli), comma shaped (vibrio), and spiral (spirilli), A, B, C, and D, respectively.

Bacteria are very simple when compared to other living things. One characteristic is that they have simple cells surrounded by a cell wall. For this reason survival functions for bacteria are simple as compared to other life forms. Bacteria can be found literally everywhere on earth and may survive in extreme conditions, including very hot, cold, acidic, and basic conditions.

One example of a simple life function carried out by bacteria is reproduction. The usual (but not the only) method of reproduction in bacteria only requires one bacterium. Most life forms require at least both a male and female to have children, right? In this method, the genetic material is copied and the bacterium simply pulls apart or divides. One cell gives rise to two *daughter* cells. In some bacteria, having children, if you will, only takes about thirty minutes. Now that's simple! This may explain why they're everywhere.

Bacteria are usually referred to by their *genus* name or both the *genus* and *species* name. Two common bacteria that infect our intestinal tract are *Salmonella* (genus) and *Escherichia coli* (genus and species), or *E. coli* for short. Some bacterial infections can cause severe complications and spread throughout the body. This is a condition known as *septicemia*. If left untreated, septicemia can lead to death. But not all bacteria are harmful. For example, if you eat yogurt, most yogurt products contain *Lactobacillus acidophilus*, a harmless bacterium that is found in the intestinal tract. *L. acidophilus* aids in digestion and destroys some disease-causing organisms.

PARASITES (THE THIEVES)

All living things need nutrition to survive. We get nutrition from the foods we eat. Parasites get nutrition the same way we do, by breaking down materials that they take in. The difference is that they *steal* nutrition by either living in or on other living things. Often they feed off of tissues and other fluids, resulting in destruction. Some parasites cause only swelling in the infected areas, while others may cause severe infections that can lead to death. As if stealing from us isn't bad enough, they can make us sick, or even kill us while they do it.

Like bacteria, parasites are also made up of cells so they are able to survive on their own. Unlike bacteria, however, they *do not* contain a cell wall. One way that scientists group parasites is by the type of cells. Parasites range in types and sizes from protozoa, which are small and made up of one cell (Fig. 3), to helminthes (worms), which are large and made up of many cells (Fig. 4). Another way to group parasites is based on their ability to move. Some parasites cannot move (nonmotile), while others can (motile).

Most get their nutrition by engulfing bacteria or other smaller protozoa. However, many may live in and get their nutrition from humans, which may result in disease. An example is *Plasmodium* (Fig. 3c), the protozoa that causes malaria. The helminthes are larger parasites that may be grouped based on their appearance (round or flat). The word *helminth* comes from the Greek for *worm*. Their complex life cycles may include an egg, larval, and several other stages.

PARASITES (PROTOZOA)[3]

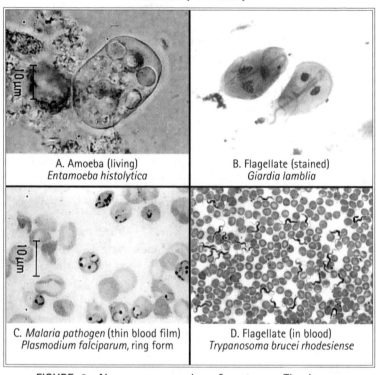

A. Amoeba (living) *Entamoeba histolytica*	B. Flagellate (stained) *Giardia lamblia*
C. *Malaria pathogen* (thin blood film) *Plasmodium falciparum*, ring form	D. Flagellate (in blood) *Trypanosoma brucei rhodesiense*

FIGURE 3. Above are examples of protozoa. The images represent examples of parasites that may cause disease in humans by inhabiting the intestines (A and B), bloodstream, and other tissues (C and D).

The most common helminth is the roundworm (Fig. 4A and 4B), which is a common cause of intestinal infection. Another common one is the tapeworm (Fig. 4C and 4D). Tapeworms can grow to be over 25 feet in length, and because they can break off like a piece of tape, each new segment is capable of becoming a new tapeworm. Parasitic worms may be found in all parts of the world and may cause infection in people of all ages.

PARASITES (HELMINTHES)[4]

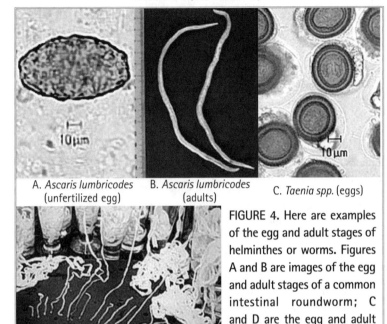

A. *Ascaris lumbricodes*
(unfertilized egg)

B. *Ascaris lumbricodes*
(adults)

C. *Taenia spp.* (eggs)

D. *Taenia spp.* (adults, living)

FIGURE 4. Here are examples of the egg and adult stages of helminthes or worms. Figures A and B are images of the egg and adult stages of a common intestinal roundworm; C and D are the egg and adult stages of a common intestinal tapeworm.

FUNGI (THE IRRITATORS)

Have you ever had an irritating rash? Chances are that at some point you have been infected by some type of fungus. Fungi can also be found almost everywhere, and many of them are important for the environment. However, many can cause problems such as allergies and a variety of infections. Many fungal infections involve the outer layers of the skin, such as nails and skin. Examples of a skin irritation caused by fungi are ringworm, jock itch, and athlete's foot. Some fungal infections involve deeper layers of the skin such as tissue and bone. Severe fungal infections occur when the fungi spread through the body. These infections often occur in individuals with compromised immune systems, such as elderly people or people with AIDS. If not treated promptly and properly, these infections may lead to severe complications and even death.

Like bacteria and parasites, fungi are also made up of cells and are able to survive on their own. Most fungi are made up of many cells; however, yeasts are an example of one-celled fungi. Fungi also get nutrition by breaking down materials that are taken in from other living things. Reproduction in fungi differs from other life forms. It often involves specialized structures called spores, and they may use them to reproduce sexually or asexually (without sex). These structures vary, and scientists use them to group fungi.

LET'S RECAP

To summarize, there are four basic types of germs that cause infectious diseases. Viruses are not true life forms because they do not have cells. They survive by using us, often resulting in sickness. Examples of common viral infections are colds and flu. Bacteria are the simplest of life forms. Remember, they have simple cells, and many can have children without a mate. Although they are the simplest, they can be the biggest nuisances because they are everywhere. Examples of common bacterial infections are wound and intestinal tract infections. Parasites are the nutrition thieves; they live in and on other living things for food. They can be very small or as large as a worm. An example of a common infection caused by parasites is intestinal tapeworms. Finally, there are fungi, complex and irritating. Fungi are responsible for a variety of infections from the outer to inner layers of our bodies. Examples are jock itch and athlete's foot.

The four types of germs that cause infectious diseases are:
- Viruses
- Bacteria
- Parasites
- Fungi

GERM TIP #1

Wow! All this information probably seems like a lot to you, and you are probably wondering how it will help you. But it is necessary information so that you may have a basic understanding of the disease-causing germs to help you prevent them. If you are going to defeat the enemy, then you must know something about it.

Chapter 2

GERMS: HOW THEY OPERATE

If you are going to defeat your enemy, it is important to know its *modus operandi*. Now that you have gained some knowledge of the germs that cause infectious diseases, let us take a look at how they operate.

We know that there are four different types of germs and that these differences are based on such things as cells, method of reproduction, and their ability to move. So the next question, then, is, how do they cause diseases? The answer is: by coming in contact with you. A germ must be contracted from a person, an object, or some other source to cause disease. In other words, germs *spread*.

HOW ARE GERMS SPREAD?

If many germs are so small that you cannot see them without special equipment, and since many of them cannot move, then how do they get around? In order to cause disease, the germs must spread and multiply. This is called the infection cycle of the germ. Germs may be spread or be *transmitted* to people in several ways. Their means of spreading is called their *mode of transmission*. They may be transmitted from human to human, from animals (or insects) to humans, or from objects to humans in five different ways: direct contact, person-to-person contact, vector-borne transmission, airborne transmission, and fecal-to-oral transmission.

Direct contact

When a person comes into physical contact with germs, this mode is known as *direct contact*. For example, if germs are located on a surface and you touch the surface, you get the germs on your hand. The germs have now made direct contact with your hand and may be able to cause infection. This is a very common mode of transmission for the viruses that cause warts.

Person-to-person contact

The mode in which a person who comes into physical contact with another person infected with germs is known as *person-to-person contact*. For example, you kiss the lips of a person who is infected with a germ, and perhaps saliva is passed. The germs have now made contact with you and may be able to cause infection. This is a very common mode of transmission for the virus that causes infectious mononucleosis, or *mono*, the "kissing disease."

Vector-borne transmission

Vector-borne transmission is the mode by which germs are transmitted via some other living thing that is a carrier, such as a mosquito or tick. For example, if a mosquito that is infected with germs bites you, then the germs are transmitted to you through the mosquito bite when it is feeding, and they pass through to your bloodstream. West Nile virus, malaria, and Lyme disease are all examples of vector-borne diseases.

Airborne transmission

Airborne transmission is the mode by which germs travel through the air and are inhaled by a person. Unlike direct or person-to-person contact, airborne transmission does not require physical contact with anything other than the air; breathing is all that is required. It may occur by breathing in respiratory droplets from coughs or sneezes from an infected person. For example, an infected person sneezes and releases viruses into the air in droplets. An innocent bystander in close proximity may become infected by inhaling the droplets. This is the mode of transmission for the viruses that cause the flu.

Fecal-to-oral transmisson

Fecal-to-oral transmission is the mode by which germs travel through the intestinal tract of a person and are released to cause infection. The germs that reside in the waste (fecal) of one person are eaten or ingested (oral) by another person. When described like that it sounds completely disgusting, but it's true. Imagine this: An infected short-order cook at a restaurant uses the restroom and does not properly wash his or her hands before preparing food. The germs may be passed from the hands of the cook to the food, then to the people who eat the food. This is often how people get sick from eating in restaurants. This is a common mode of transmission for *germs* that reside in the gut or gastrointestinal tract—the germs that cause diarrhea.

GERM TIP #2:

There are five ways that germs are spread to cause infectious diseases:
1. Direct contact
2. Person-to-person contact
3. Vector-borne transmission
4. Airborne transmission
5. Fecal-to-oral transmission

WHAT IS AN INFECTION?

So now that we know what germs are and how they are spread, let's learn what each germ does to cause an infection. Of course, we will begin with my favorite, viruses. Once a virus is transmitted to a person, it gets inside to make contact with cells. The infection cycle begins when the virus attaches itself to cells. After attachment to the cell, viruses begin to use the materials within the cell to duplicate themselves. Remember, viruses invade and use the cells in our bodies to survive. They are released from the cell to go on to attach to and enter other nearby cells. Infection occurs as a result of newly formed viruses spreading to many cells.

Bacteria and fungi often infect specialized groups of cells in our bodies called tissues. The skin, intestines, and kidneys are all examples of tissues that can be infected. The infection cycles of bacteria and fungi are quite different. They often travel through the bloodstream of our bodies and associate themselves with the tissues. Once they have found their resting place, they begin to grow and multiply. You may remember that many bacteria can do this very quickly. Infection occurs as a result of many of these germs becoming associated with specific tissues in our bodies.

Parasites also attack specific tissues in our bodies. They locate their place of residence and begin to feed off of the tissue. They steal nutrients from the cells of the tissue they infect and can often cause major destruction. The infection cycle of these germs ends when they are cleared or released from the bodies of their host to infect other individuals, thus beginning the infection cycle again.

HOW DO GERMS MAKE US SICK?

Sickness occurs when our bodies try to destroy the germs that infect us. The human body is an awesome creation by God. It was designed with a defense mechanism known as the immune system that has the sole purpose of protecting it from invasion and injury. Our immune system can recognize when there is something present in our body that does not belong. Think about it as you would a combat situation. Once the enemy is recognized, our immune system does everything in its power to destroy or remove the enemy from our body. Our body has two types of immunity to protect us from disease: nonspecific immunity and specific immunity. Nonspecific immunity involves methods of protection from all germs, while specific immunity is targeted against a specific type of germ.

Nonspecific immunity

Our nonspecific immune system works very much like doors on a home. When closed, the doors keep invaders from entering. So our nonspecific immune system acts as a barrier to prevent germs from infecting our bodies. Our bodies have four types of barriers that are used to protect us from harmful germs: physical, physiologic, chemical, and cells.

Our skin is the first physical barrier of our nonspecific immune system. It is comprised of an outer and inner layer. The outer layer contains tightly packed cells, which make it very difficult for germs to enter our bodies. This is why when we get a cut or scrape we should immediately clean and cover it. It is like fixing a broken window at your home. It prevents access to the inside. The skin's inner layer contains glands that secrete acidic materials, a condition that many germs don't like.

A second example of a physical barrier is mucous membranes. These are the cells that line and cover many organs in our bodies. The lining of our respiratory tract, for example, is covered with short hairs that aid in trapping and moving germs. Saliva, tears, and mucus are all secretions from mucous membranes. They act to remove germs from our bodies. This explains why some infections involve sneezing, watery eyes, and a runny nose. They are all ways to remove germs from our bodies.

The conditions inside our bodies, or *physiologic* conditions, also act as a barrier. Our normal body temperature is favorable for many germs. However, when we become infected, our body temperature becomes elevated (fever), making conditions less favorable for germs. Another example of a physiologic barrier is pH. The pH determines if something is either an acid or a base. Our skin and the inside of our stomachs are very acidic. Many germs cannot grow in an acidic environment, so this condition provides general protection from them.

If germs are able to evade the body's physical and physiologic barriers, then there are still chemical barriers left to contend with. Our bodies contain many proteins and other chemicals that act to kill germs. One example is complement, which is a group of proteins that circulate throughout our bodies. When germs, such as bacteria, enter our bodies, complement proteins are activated. The end result is destruction of the bacteria. Also, there are proteins in our bodies that are used to help cells stop the spread of viruses.

Finally, there are the cells. Cells in our bodies may also destroy germs and other foreign materials that enter our bodies. They do it by engulfing and degrading the material. It's kind of like eating them. Special cells in our bodies are able to identify germs, and they simply devour them. Now that's protection!

When your nonspecific immune system is working hard to protect you, you begin to feel sick. Your body temperature rises to try to destroy the germs infecting you, causing you to develop a fever. Your body attempts to remove the germs by trapping them in the short hairs in your nose and secreting mucus to remove them from your body. The result is a runny nose, coughing, and watery eyes. Mucus is secreted in your throat to trap germs, and you develop a sore throat. You swallow some of the germs trapped in the mucus in your throat, which are released into your stomach, a very acidic environment. You even experience symptoms to remove the germs in saliva, like sneezing. Do you now see how the symptoms we feel when we are sick can actually be a *good* thing? It is our immune system working to kill and remove the germs from our body. Although the nonspecific immune system works to defend us from *general* invasion by germs, sometimes it is necessary to have a more *specific* method of defense.

Specific immunity

There are distinct differences between nonspecific and specific immunity. First, nonspecific immunity responds to *all* germs, while specific immunity occurs when we come into contact with a *specific type* of germ. It is targeted toward that germ *only*. Second, while nonspecific immunity occurs immediately after exposure, specific immunity takes time to get the maximal protection. Third, specific immunity involves memory. Your immune system meets the germ once and remembers it the next time it sees it. There are two types of specific immunity: humoral and cell mediated.

Humoral immunity involves white blood cells called B cells. These cells produce antibodies, the proteins that target the specific germs. Antibodies bind to the germs and inactivate them. Afterwards, the B cells produce more antibodies that can react to the same type (specific) of germ. The next time you are exposed to it, there will be lots of B cells that remember (memory B cells) the germ and can respond quickly. This is the maximum response and explains the time. It is the response after the first exposure to the germ.

Cell-mediated immunity involves white blood cells called T cells. One type of T cells is killer T cells. These cells are able to direct the destruction of other cells, such as cells that are infected with germs. When T cells identify cells that have been infected with viruses or bacteria, they send signals to those cells that help them die. The infected cell does not try to survive. Since the germs can multiply, the cell will cooperate to prevent further spread of the germs to other cells. It's as if the T cell says to the infected cell, "Hey, you are infected by a germ, and you must be destroyed," and the infected cell agrees. It is a true sacrifice for the greater good of the rest of the body. The other type of T cells is helper T cells.

These cells send signals to other T cells and B cells to "help" them to do their jobs. Both types of T cells *mediate* the destruction of germs.

All of this explains why we feel so awful when we are infected with germs. When our immune system is working, it also causes pain, redness, and swelling to occur at the site of infection. This is a condition commonly referred to as inflammation. Sneezing, coughing, watery eyes, vomiting, and diarrhea are also ways of releasing germs in bodily fluids. We may feel awful, but it actually helps us to clear the infection. Unfortunately, when we have these symptoms, we are releasing the germs into the environment for others to come into contact with, ingest, or inhale. This is why germs are continuously spread and make people sick.

GERM TIP #3: Germs make us sick by triggering our immune system. Some effects are:
- Elevated body temperature (fever)
- Fluid discharge (sneezing, coughing, watery eyes, diarrhea, vomiting)
- Heat, pain, redness, and swelling (inflammation)

Understanding how germs spread will help you to decrease the risk of becoming infected. It is truly amazing when you think about how our bodies are awesome creations of God. He equipped our bodies with not just one, but two immune systems. One provides a general protection from all germs by using different types of barriers, while the second system memorizes a specific germ and targets it. Our bodies truly are remarkable, complex machines.

As amazing as our immune system is, germs are "smart," if you will. They are still able to get in and cause disease. They have found ways to get past every barrier and defense. Some of these germs have made media headlines. In the next chapter, I will "disarm" some of the fear raised by those germs.

Chapter 3

GERMS IN THE MEDIA

"FDA Recalls Bad Beef." "West Nile Virus Claims Thousands of Lives." "SARS Reaches Epidemic Proportions." These are bogus headlines, but they're not completely unrealistic. Disease names such as SARS, anthrax, mad cow disease, and West Nile virus infection have become almost commonplace in our everyday vocabulary because the media has given them so much attention. The interesting thing is that the germs that have been media headliners are the least common of all infectious diseases. Ironically, infectious diseases that have the greatest public health impact rarely get media attention. It would be impossible to write a book about infectious diseases without mentioning the germs that have become famous in recent years. Allow me to introduce to you the "stars" of the germ world.

MEET ANTHRAX—THE "SLEEPING BEAUTY"

Shortly after the 9/11 terrorist attacks, we became vulnerable to another form of terrorism—bioterrorism. Nobody would have imagined that such a small agent could ignite such large-scale fear.

Anthrax is a disease caused by the bacterium *Bacillus anthracis*. One interesting feature of these bacteria is that they form spores, cells that are dormant or "asleep" until conditions cause them to "wake up." Anthrax is not spread by person-to-person contact but rather by direct contact or inhalation of spores. This mode of transmission along with the effects of the disease is what causes this disease to be of great public health importance.

The CDC classifies anthrax as a category A (top priority) agent. This means that it can be easily spread, can result in high death rates, and has the potential for major public health impact. Such an agent may spread across a large area, and it will require a great deal of planning to protect the public from its effects. Other examples of category A agents are smallpox and botulism. Category B agents are moderately easy to spread and may result in moderate death rates. Examples of category B agents are food safety threats such as *Samonella* and *E. coli*. Category C agents are germs that can be engineered for mass destruction in the future. They are the third highest priority agents. Anthrax can be used as a biological weapon, as we witnessed in the United States in 2001. Anthrax was spread as a powder on letters delivered through the postal service. As a result, twenty-two people became infected.

Diseases and symptoms

There are three types of anthrax infections: skin, gastrointestinal, and lungs. The symptoms for all three types of infections may occur within seven days of contact with the bacteria. Skin infections are transmitted by direct contact. Symptoms first occur as a sore that soon develops into a blister. The blister will then develop into a skin ulcer. Infections of the gastrointestinal tract occur through direct contact such as eating undercooked meat from an infected animal. The symptoms include fever, bloody diarrhea, stomach pain, and nausea. Lung infections are transmitted through inhalation of bacterial spores. The first symptoms are similar to other respiratory tract infections such as colds and flu and may also include fever, sore throat, and muscle aches. Later symptoms include chest pains, shortness of breath, and tiredness. If a person experiences cold- or flu-like symptoms, he shouldn't panic and run to his doctor. Almost all cold or flu symptoms are simply that, a cold or the flu.

Treatment

All three forms of anthrax are treated with antibiotics, and success is usually dependent on how early the treatment begins. Skin infections are usually not severe. Even if untreated, 80 percent do not end in death. Gastrointestinal and lung infections are far more severe. From one-fourth to one-half of persons with gastrointestinal infections die. Of the cases that occurred in the United States in 2001 that were lung infections, approximately 50 percent resulted in death.[1]

Prevention

So what can a person do to prevent becoming infected with anthrax? There is a vaccine for anthrax, but it is not yet available for general public use. Those who have been at highest risk for infection include postal workers, military personnel, laboratory personnel, and persons who worked in contaminated areas. These people received the vaccine, which was of limited supply.

Although there was a great deal of media coverage for anthrax, there is no need to be fearful of contracting the disease. Since 2001, the CDC has been working very hard to prepare for possible anthrax attacks. Laboratories are prepared to rapidly detect the bacteria that cause the disease. Additionally, safety evaluations are routinely conducted to prevent the possible spread of the bacteria.

BAD BEEF (AKA MAD COW DISEASE)

Another germ that has achieved "star power" and notoriety is bovine spongiform encephalopathy (BSE), commonly referred to as mad cow disease. BSE is a neurological disorder of cattle. This disease is believed to be caused by a different type of infectious agent, which is found in abnormally folded proteins called prions. It was first identified in 1996 in the United Kingdom where large outbreaks in cattle occurred, resulting in over 183,000 cases by 2003. It has since been identified in at least twenty European countries, Canada, Japan, and Israel. It is clear that one factor that contributes to the spread of BSE among cattle is feeding them BSE-contaminated meat-and-bone meal. In December 2003 the first laboratory confirmed case of BSE occurred in the United States in the state of Washington.[2] An investigation revealed that the infected cow was imported into the United States from Canada. Since then the levels of concern about protecting the United States food supply remain high.

Disease and symptoms

The disease in humans is believed to be caused by a variant form of the neurological disorder Creutzfeldt-Jakob disease (vCJD). Classical Creutzfeldt-Jakob disease (CJD) is a fatal neurological disorder. Most people die within one year of the onset of disease. In contrast to the classical CJD, vCJD displays a delayed onset of symptoms, and the illness lasts at least six months. Also, vCJD typically affects young people, whereas the average age of death among CJD patients is sixty-eight years old. As of December 2003, a total of 153 cases of vCJD had been reported, with 143 identified in the United Kingdom. Almost all of these cases involved exposure during the months of the cattle outbreaks. There have been no cases reported outside of a country where BSE was occurring. In 2002, the CDC reported a case of vCJD in a Florida resident who was born and grew up in the United Kingdom. The CDC claims that the risk of BSE to human health in the United States is low.

Here are some symptoms of mad cow disease that you can identify:

- Illness usually occuring in young people; the average age, twenty-nine years old
- Sensory symptoms at the time of illness (i.e. vision, balance)
- Psychiatric symptoms at the time of illness (i.e. delusions, mood swings)
- Symptoms continuing for at least six months

Prevention and surveillance

The question: is our food safe? The answer: yes. The Department of Health and Human Services (DHHS) has developed a four-component plan for BSE: protection, surveillance, research, and oversight.

1. **Protection**—The Food and Drug Administration (FDA) has placed restrictions on the importation of cattle, goats, sheep, and other products from many European and other countries to prevent BSE from entering the United States. The FDA also instituted a ruminant feed ban that became effective in 1997.
2. **Surveillance**—The Centers for Disease Control and Prevention (CDC) monitors the number of cases by analyzing data compiled from death certificates

gathered by the National Center for Health Statistics. Additionally, the CDC collects data and investigates reports of possible cases of the disease.

3. **Research**—The National Institutes of Health (NIH) conducts research to obtain an understanding of the germs—prions—that cause the disease.

4. **Oversight**—The Department of Health and Human Services (DHHS) reviews the data and control measures implemented by each of these agencies. This information is used to develop policies that protect public health.

So as you see, before the food ends up on your dinner table, there is a strict criterion to ensure the public's safety.

INTRODUCING SARS

Severe acute respiratory syndrome (SARS), a disease caused by a coronavirus, has been one of the biggest scares of recent history. As with other respiratory illnesses, it is transmitted by close person-to-person contact with an infected person *via* respiratory droplets. The virus can also be spread when people have direct contact with a contaminated surface and then touch their nose, mouth, or eyes. It is also possible that airborne transmission of the SARS virus occurs. The first case was reported in Asia in February 2003. If you were watching the news, you probably remember seeing Asian people walking around wearing surgical masks. Shortly after the first case was reported in Asia, a global outbreak occurred when the virus spread to several countries in Asia, Europe, North America, and South America. The World Health Organization (WHO) reported a total of over 8,000 cases *worldwide* resulting in 774 deaths.[3] Only 8 laboratory confirmed cases were reported in the United States, none of which resulted in death.

Disease and symptoms

As the name suggests, the disease is a severe respiratory illness. Initial symptoms include fever, headache, and discomfort sometimes accompanied by mild respiratory symptoms. A small percentage of patients also experience diarrhea. Most patients develop a dry cough between two and seven days after onset, which may then develop into pneumonia. Patients are believed to be contagious only after the onset of symptoms.

Treatment

Currently there is no known SARS-specific antiviral treatment. Patients generally received the same treatment that would be given to people with other forms of atypical pneumonia.

Prevention

The best prevention method of SARS would be the same as with other respiratory illnesses. You should avoid prolonged close contact with people who are sick, especially avoiding contact with respiratory droplets (when a person coughs or sneezes).

Surveillance

Again, there is no need to fear. Since the global outbreak, several rapid diagnostic tests for the SARS virus have been developed. What does this mean? It means that infection with this virus can be diagnosed very quickly. Rapid detection is the key to intervention. It allows public health officials to immediately implement plans to prevent further spread of the disease. These control measures began during the global outbreak of 2003. The CDC, WHO, and other groups worked collaboratively to investigate and control the spread of SARS. Medical experts and support staff were provided for suspected SARS cases. Laboratory assistance was provided for state and local health departments, and health alert notices were distributed for travelers. Today, the CDC works with other federal agencies and local and state health departments to assist in the rapid detection and response to SARS infections.

THE "BUZZ" ON THE WEST NILE VIRUS

Most people love summertime. Daylight lasts longer, so you can do fun activities. You can go swimming, play ball, enjoy picnics, take long walks, and dodge mosquitoes. Seriously though, mosquitoes are carriers of a virus that can cause a serious illness known as the West Nile virus (WNV).

West Nile virus was first isolated in 1937 from an adult woman in the West Nile district of Uganda. In 1957 it became recognized as a cause of severe meningitis and encephalitis in an outbreak in Israel. It was first reported in the United States in 1999. Since then it has become a great public health concern because it has resulted in significant illness. WNV is now the cause of epidemics in North America and parts of Europe in the summer and continuing until fall. In 2004 a total of 2,470 cases of human WNV infections were reported to the CDC.[4] The virus has now been reported in Africa, Europe, Asia, the Middle East, and Oceana.

The most common way for WNV to spread to humans is from the bite of an infected mosquito. Mosquitoes become infected by feeding on infected birds. The virus has also been known to spread to humans via organ transplants and blood transfusions. There has also been one reported case of transmission from mother-to-child and one case of transmission associated with breast milk. WNV has not been shown to be transmitted through direct person-to-person contact.

Disease and symptoms

WNV affects the central nervous system; however; approximately 80 percent of people infected with WNV show no symptoms at all. For people who do develop symptoms, they usually occur between three and fourteen days *after* they have been bitten by an infected mosquito. Up to 20 percent of people infected will have mild symptoms that are typical of viral infections, including fever, nausea, vomiting, body aches, swollen lymph nodes, and rashes. These symptoms can last from a few days to up to a few weeks.[5] It is reported that one in one hundred fifty people infected may develop severe symptoms, which can include a high fever, muscle weakness, and even vision loss. Symptoms affecting the nervous system may include disorientation, tremors, numbness, coma, and paralysis. Neurological symptoms may be permanent. People over fifty have a greater risk of becoming ill from WNV infections because they are less likely to take the necessary precautions.

Treatment

Unfortunately, there is no specific treatment for infection with WNV at the time of this writing. The symptoms of mild infections are treated just as any other viral infections. Most people who experience severe symptoms are hospitalized.

Prevention

The best way to prevent WNV infection is to prevent mosquito bites by:

- Applying insect repellents containing DEET to your skin and clothes
- Trying to stay inside during the times when mosquitoes are most active (usually dusk and dawn)
- Wearing long sleeves and pants when you are in environments with lots of mosquitoes
- Making sure you remove mosquito breeding sites such as containers of standing water around your home
- Repairing all screen doors and windows at your home

Surveillance

People have become more fearful of mosquitoes each year since the news of West Nile virus infections. There is no need to fear. Following the simple prevention methods described above should greatly reduce your risk of becoming infected. Also, be assured that the CDC is doing everything possible to support WNV surveillance by opening new laboratories for WNV testing. There has also been funding provided to support the development of rapid diagnostic tests for WNV, and a nationwide electronic database has been established to monitor the number of WNV cases.

LET'S RECAP

Although the diseases associated with these germs can be devastating, the risk of becoming infected with them is relatively low. Even as of this writing, there were other germs that became the newest "stars," and the content in this chapter would be endless!

These germs do not impact public health nearly as much as many of the other germs that you will read about in the next chapters. I hope that the information discussed in this chapter has relieved some of your fears of becoming infected with these germs. You don't need to drastically change your lifestyle.

UNIT 2

GERMS AND INFECTIOUS DISEASES

Chapter 4

COLDS AND FLU

Can you count the number of times you or someone in your family has been sick with a cold? Don't try. I know the answer to that question. Colds are probably the most common of all infectious diseases, hence the name *common cold*. What about the flu? It is equally common. Each year we dread the countdown to the approaching flu season. These two diseases are so common that they have become marketable. Advertisements for cold and flu medicines are appropriately timed between back-to-school and Christmas sales. Why is it that people know the symptoms and time of year they occur, but very little else that is true about these two diseases? Since they are the most common infectious diseases, I would like to begin by clarifying some common misconceptions about them.

COLDS

The myths

Many people have the misconception that colds are caused by cold weather and that not dressing properly for the weather conditions will lead to the illness. A second misconception is that a person must be ill or have a weakened immune system to be susceptible to colds. Each is a myth about how people contract colds. It is very important to seek the truth in all things, particularly in areas that affect your health and well-being. The Bible emphasizes the importance of seeking the truth. (See Psalm 25:5.)

The truth

First, colds are caused by viruses. In order to get sick from the viruses that cause colds, you must come into contact with them. They must attach to your cells and multiply within your cells to cause infection. Although not dressing properly for the weather conditions is probably not a good idea, there is no direct evidence that a person can contract a cold because of it. Second, a person need not have a weakened immune system to be susceptible to infections with cold viruses. In a study involving healthy adults, 95 percent became infected when cold viruses were administered through the nose.[1] Of those, a large percentage developed symptoms associated with the common cold.

Germs

More than two hundred viruses are known to cause colds, and to date, there is no vaccine. There are so many different types or *strains* of cold viruses that it is very difficult to develop a vaccine to provide protection from them all. Below is a list of some of the viruses that have been associated with the common cold. For many of those listed, several strains have been identified.

Some viruses associated with the common cold are:

- Rhinoviruses
- Respiratory syncytial virus
- Human parainfluenza virus
- Coronaviruses
- Adenoviruses
- Coxsackieviruses
- Orthomyxoviruses

Transmission and symptoms

Sneezing, coughing, runny nose, sore throat, and headache are all symptoms associated with the common cold. A cold is an infection of the upper respiratory tract, which includes the nose and throat. Unlike what many people think about the transmission of colds, the viruses that cause colds are usually transmitted by direct contact with the hands. The hands then touch the mouth, nose, or eyes, and the virus multiplies in the nose. The symptoms are probably the result of the body's immune response to the virus. This causes inflammation in the lining of the nose, resulting in sneezing and a blocked, runny nose. Fluid may drain from the nose to the throat, causing soreness, and from the back of the throat to the chest, causing coughing. The symptoms may last from two to fourteen days.

Studies suggest that people are more likely to transmit viruses and are more contagious on the second to fourth days of infections.

This is the time when the concentration of virus in nasal secretions is greatest. It takes only a few days after infection for illness to develop, but it usually goes away within a week. In some cases, colds may lead to secondary bacterial infections of the middle ear or sinuses, requiring treatment with antibiotics.

Seasonality

Most colds in the United States occur during the fall and winter months. The incidence for colds increases slowly beginning in late August and early September and remains high until the spring months. There are possible explanations for the seasonality of colds. First, most schools commence the school year in August or September, depending upon the region. Students are exposed to other students who may carry the virus, and so begins the "cold season." Another possible explanation is that the virus can spread easily among people because people are more likely to stay indoors during cold weather.

THE FLU

The myths

Many people have the same misconceptions about the flu as they do for colds. One is the belief that the flu can be contracted from cold weather conditions. Another is that you must be sick to be susceptible to the flu. There is also the belief that the symptoms of a cold can become so severe that it can develop into or become the flu.

The truth

The flu is also a respiratory infection caused by viruses. Just as with cold viruses, you must be exposed to the flu virus to become infected. It is not transmitted via cold weather, nor is it necessary to be sick to become infected. Unless a person is infected with both cold and flu viruses, it is unlikely that a cold will develop into the flu. It is more likely that the symptoms of a severe cold and the flu are so similar that it is difficult for many people to distinguish between the two diseases.

Almost every winter flu viruses cause epidemics leading to both the hospitalization and death of many people worldwide. The CDC estimates that 10–20 percent of Americans are infected with the flu virus each year. Of those, an average of 114,000 is hospitalized each year for complications associated with the infection. The most startling reports, however, are related to the number of deaths that occur each year: an estimated 36,000 Americans die each year from complications of the flu.

Germs

There are three types of viruses that cause the flu: influenza types A, B, and C. Influenza type A is further classified into two groups based on their types of surface proteins that are recognized by our immune systems. Influenza types A and B viruses are the most common cause of disease each year. Influenza type C causes less severe respiratory infections and is usually not involved in epidemics. The type A influenza virus has also been found in animals, including birds, pigs, and whales.

Transmission and symptoms

The mode of transmission for flu viruses is respiratory droplets from sneezes and coughs. An infected person may sneeze or cough, and droplets carrying the virus may get on the mouth or nose of a person in close proximity. This gives the virus access to the cells of the respiratory tract, thus causing illness. Adults may be contagious before symptoms and are capable of spreading the germs for up to seven days after symptoms appear. Children may be contagious for several days before the onset of symptoms and may be contagious for ten days or more afterwards. Persons who are immune compromised may spread viruses for months.

Symptoms from the flu are usually far more severe than a cold. They also occur very quickly after infection. In addition to the common cold symptoms, flu symptoms include high fever (above 102° F), headaches, body aches, muscle aches, and tiredness. Sometimes people with the flu contract secondary infections, causing complications. Some examples are bacterial pneumonia, ear and sinus infections, and worsening of long-term chronic illnesses. If severe, the infection may be treated with prescribed antiviral drugs. There are several types of antiviral treatments for flu infections, but they must be prescribed within the first couple of days after the onset of illness. Therefore, it is very important to seek medical attention early if symptoms become severe or are complicated by secondary infections. The CDC recommends that parents should look out for the following warning signs in children.[2]

- Fast breathing or trouble breathing
- Bluish skin color
- Not drinking enough fluids
- Not waking up or not interacting
- Being so irritable that the child does not want to be held
- Flu-like symptoms improve but then return with fever and worse cough
- Fever with a rash

If these signs are observed, seek medical attention for your child immediately.

Risk groups

Although it is recommended that everyone get annual immunizations if possible, there are certain groups that are more likely to have serious health problems if they get the flu. The first risk group is children between the ages of six months and twenty-three months; the flu vaccine has not been approved for children under six months old. The CDC reports that recent studies have shown that even healthy children under two years old are more likely to have severe health complications from the flu, even death.[3] People sixty-five years of age and older, especially those who live in primary-care facilities, are also more likely to have severe health complications from the flu. Another risk group is people who have underlying long-term illnesses, including diabetes, heart disease, and lung disease, and people who are immune compromised. Other risk groups include people who are caregivers for these groups or in health-care facilities. Indeed, clinical studies have shown that those at risk for heart attacks, who receive their annual flu shot, are less likely to suffer future heart attacks.[4]

Specific prevention of the flu

As with the cold, there is no cure for the flu. There are, however, some specific measures that can be taken to prevent the flu. Vaccination is an effective way to prevent illness caused by the flu virus. One challenge with vaccination with the influenza virus is that the virus changes quite often, resulting in new strains of influenza viruses. Vaccines are the actual germ or part of the germ that our immune system recognizes; they work because of our body's specific immunity. (Remember our discussion in chapter two?) We are only protected from the germ that we have been vaccinated with; therefore, if the germ changes, our immune system will not recognize it. This is why annual immunizations are necessary to prevent infection. Each year a new vaccine is developed, and it includes strains that are currently in circulation.

A second way to prevent infection with influenza viruses is to take antiviral drugs. There are a few antiviral drugs that are available for prevention of the flu; examples are amantadine and rimantadine. Of course, please consult your physician before using this approach. Also, they are prescribed early in the course of the infection, so you must see a physician immediately after symptoms appear.

GENERAL PREVENTION OF COLDS AND FLU

The Bible provides specific instructions for how to prevent the spread of infection. It specifically describes what sickness is (discharge, i.e. fluid or mucus) and addresses the importance of washing (bathing) to prevent infection. (See Leviticus 15:5, 7, 11, 13.)

One preventive measure described is to not touch things that sick people have touched, and if so, wash. A second is do not touch or have contact with a sick person, and if so, wash. A third is to isolate yourself for seven days if you are sick. If you recall, this is the period of time for which the viruses are contagious. These same preventive measures mentioned in the Bible are now suggested by health-care professionals for cold and flu viruses. You may see now why I mentioned that the health sciences are just now beginning to catch up with the Bible.

To prevent infection with cold and flu viruses:
- Avoid contact with people that are sick.
- Wash your hands often, especially after coming in contact with objects handled by someone sick.
- Avoid touching your face when you around people who are sick.

GERM TIP #4

Why is the information in this chapter important? It is important because more people are affected by colds and flu—respiratory infections—than any of the other types of infectious diseases. You are far more likely to become infected with a cold or flu virus than any of the germs mentioned in the previous unit. Really, anthrax is not responsible for the death of thirty-six thousand Americans each year. However, no one is particularly interested in discussing these germs in the media unless there are some major differences observed (for example, bird flu) or something happens to create a panic (for example, vaccine shortage). So, if you don't hear about them in the media, how can you be assured that these respiratory viruses aren't hospitalizing and killing people on an even larger scale? How can you feel safe?

Surveillance

The good news is that there is national surveillance of respiratory diseases such as colds and flu in the United States. Know that health professionals, governmental health departments, the CDC, and other agencies are working together to ensure the public's safety and health.

To conclude, colds and flu are very common respiratory infections that probably have a greater effect on public health than any other disease. The take-home message is that these diseases can affect people of all ages, and there is no cure for either of them. Fortunately, applying the simple preventive practices described in this chapter can greatly reduce the risks of infection.

Chapter 5

PNEUMONIA

It feels like a cold, but it's not; it's far worse. Chest pains, persistent coughing, tiredness, and an awful headache that won't go away are also a part of it. It's pneumonia, another common illness of the respiratory tract. It arises from infection and inflammation of the lungs. It can happen to people of all ages and is caused by a variety of germs. An estimated two to five million cases occur each year in the United States, with five hundred thousand pneumonia-related hospitalizations. Often outbreaks occur in crowded institutional settings such as colleges and jails. Some germs that cause pneumonia become invasive, resulting in death in 14 percent of hospitalized adults.[1] Pneumonia is similar to the flu in that it is transmitted in the same manner and it can cause a wide spectrum of illnesses. There are, however, some very distinct differences between the two diseases, and it is helpful to have knowledge of them both.

GERMS

Unlike the flu, which is caused by a virus, pneumonia is most commonly caused by a variety of bacteria and usually only one virus. (See Table 1.) The risk groups and severity of symptoms are determined by the type of germ that causes infection. No matter what the age group, it is an awful infection that we most certainly want to try to prevent whenever possible.

TRANSMISSION AND SYMPTOMS

Similar to the flu, pneumonia is transmitted by person-to-person contact via respiratory droplets from secretions in the nose and saliva. Mild symptoms include cough, malaise, and headache. Other symptoms include:

Table 1: Common Germs That Cause Pneumonia and Risk Groups[2]	
BACTERIA	**RISK GROUPS**
Chlamydia pneumoniae	All ages, most common among school-age children
Haemophilus influenzae serotype B	1980–1990—Infants and young children, household contacts, day-care classmates; routine vaccination has decreased incidence.
Mycoplasma pneumoniae	Persons of all ages, but rarely children less than five years old, most often associated with outbreaks
Streptococcus pneumoniae	Alcoholics, people with sickle-cell disease, elderly, and immune-compromised persons. Drug-resistant forms occur in groups where there is frequent use of antibiotics.
VIRUS	**RISK GROUPS**
Human Parainfluenza Virus	Elderly and immune-compromised persons

- Sharp or stabbing chest pain
- Shortness of breath
- Rapid, shallow breathing
- Loss of appetite

Once infected by the germs that cause pneumonia, a variety of tissues may be affected, resulting in inflammation. Included among these are inflammation of the sinuses (sinusitis), the bronchi (bronchitis), and the larynx (laryngitis). Some bacteria may even infect tissues around the heart (peritonitis) and joints (arthritis). In severe cases the bacteria may spread and infect parts of the brain and nervous system (meningitis). Pneumonia is a very serious disease and should be treated immediately after diagnosis. It is also very important to take precautionary measures to prevent the spread of pneumonia to others.

PREVENTION

If the cause is bacterial, then your physician might prescribe an antibiotic. Because the bacteria that cause pneumonia are spread by people via respiratory droplets, the best way to prevent infection is to avoid contact with people who are sick. The symptoms of pneumonia are very obvious, so it is unlikely that a person will be infected for very long unknowingly. The best preventative measures you can take are to wash your hands frequently and avoid contact with respiratory droplets. Check with your physician about getting vaccinated if you are in a high-risk category, such as the elderly and people with chronic conditions.

Some important things to remember about pneumonia:
- Unlike colds and flu, it is often caused by bacteria and may be treated with antibiotics.
- It is transmitted by close person-to-person contact via respiratory droplets.
- Seek medical attention if severe; bacterial infections may spread to other tissues.

GERM TIP #5

SURVEILLANCE

As with the flu, there is comfort in knowing that patterns of pneumonia infections are also monitored each year in the United States. The CDC has coordinated surveillance systems for many of the germs that cause pneumonia.

Having discussed the more common respiratory infections—colds, flu, and pneumonia—let's take a closer look at two common childhood illnesses: ear and throat infections.

Chapter 6

EAR AND THROAT INFECTIONS

Some childhood illnesses seem unavoidable. Earaches and sore throats are great examples. If you have children or work with children, then I'm sure that at some time they have suffered from one, if not both, of these illnesses. For some children these infections occur frequently. So often, in fact, that their parents don't take them to see a doctor. Even if a child gets these illnesses often, it is wise to see a professional. Earaches and sore throats are often signs of an infection. Infections always have the possibility of becoming complicated and causing severe illness if not treated properly.

This chapter provides information about infections of the ears and throat. Ear infections are especially common among young children. Infections of the throat affect most people by the time they reach adulthood, but some of the germs that cause these infections may also be carried on the skin and not cause symptoms. Both may also lead to severe complications if not treated properly. The Bible explains that having knowledge and good understanding adds favor and health to your life.

> The law of the wise is a fountain of life, to depart from the snares of death. Good understanding giveth favour: but the way of transgressors is hard. Every prudent man dealeth with knowledge: but a fool layeth open his folly. A wicked messenger falleth into mischief: but a faithful ambassador is health.
> —PROVERBS 13:14–17

Because they are so common and can lead to complications, it is important to have knowledge of these diseases.

EAR INFECTIONS

I feel most qualified as a parent, not a microbiologist, to write about ear infections, and I would like to share my experience with you. My daughter was under two years old when her ear infections began. I always knew what the problem was because the symptoms were the same. It started with her hands on her ear. It didn't matter what she was doing—eating, playing, even napping—her hand would frequently gravitate toward her ear as if it were a reflex. Soon afterwards, she would become groggy. After a day or two of hand action, she would say, "Mommy, my ear hurts." If she were not seen by a doctor immediately, by the evening she would develop a fever. The pain would be unbearable for her. The doctors always said the same thing, "She has an ear infection." Each time they prescribed antibiotics—sometimes the same type, sometimes a different type. The ear infections were frequent, at least four each year, and often they were concurrent. This continued until she was about five years old. Two doctors recommended that she have tubes put in her ears to decrease the frequency of the infections.

I am sure that many parents and caregivers of young children can identify with my story. The three years of frequent ear infections were a very difficult time for my family. As a parent, I felt helpless because I thought there was nothing that I could do to prevent them. It hurt me to watch my daughter suffer. Also, I did not want to continuously give her antibiotics. We thank God that she made it through this period with no permanent damage to her ears. She no longer gets ear infections, and she has excellent hearing.

The cause and symptoms

I started to notice a pattern when my daughter would get ear infections. It always seemed to follow a cold, congestion, or respiratory symptoms. I remember not being satisfied with the answers the doctors gave me about the cause. So, I began reading about it. I learned that ear infections take place in the middle ear, an area of the ear that contains air and sits behind the eardrum. The eustachian tube connects the middle ear to the nose and acts to equalize pressure in the middle ear. In children, the eustachian tube is shorter and less slanted than in adults. This allows bacteria easy access to this area. During a respiratory infection, the nasal canal and eustachian tube become swollen and congested. Since you understand how infection occurs, you can guess what the result is. Yes, inflammation. The middle ear becomes filled with fluid, resulting in pain and sometimes temporary loss of hearing. Fever often accompanies ear infections because the body is trying to fight it.

There are other types of ear infections that are more severe. One occurs when the middle ear is filled with fluid, for long periods of time. It is called otitis media with effusion and occurs when the eustachian tube is not functioning properly. This condition does not require a previous ear infection to occur. The second type is called chronic otitis media. It occurs when an ear infection continues for more than two weeks. Both conditions can become severe because the middle ear and ear drum may be damaged. The result can be permanent hearing loss.

Treatment

Antibiotics are the prescribed treatment for most ear infections. They should be taken exactly as prescribed to completely clear the infection. If the symptoms persist and infections recur frequently, it may be necessary to see an ear, nose, and throat (ENT) specialist. Fever reducers and pain relievers are also recommended sometimes to help a child feel more comfortable. Many parents are concerned about permanent loss of hearing. If medications are taken as prescribed, these risks are minimized.

Prevention

- In newborn children, breastfeeding passes protective antibodies to the child.
- Decrease exposure to people with respiratory illnesses.
- Follow preventive measures described for respiratory illnesses in previous chapters.
- Keep your child away from secondhand smoke.
- If symptoms occur, always see a physician immediately to decrease the risks of complications and long-term damage.
- Talk to the doctors and ask questions.

As I reflect on this time, I am sure that I did not ask the doctors enough questions. I would like to encourage parents to ask questions when their children suffer from any type of infection. If you do not completely understand or feel that you have not received enough information, ask the doctor to clarify and explain. Doctors have the call of healing on their lives. Most are more than happy to take the time to help parents have a complete understanding of the child's illness.

THROAT INFECTIONS

Now that we have learned about the causes, symptoms, treatments, and prevention for ear infections, it's time to move on to the throat. I know that I don't need to provide statistics to inform you how often people get sore throats. Sore throats are often symptoms of respiratory illnesses such as colds, flu, and pneumonia. However, sometimes germs actually infect and cause disease in the throat. Following is information about two diseases that specifically affect the throat—strep throat and "mono."

STREP THROAT

Germs

There are several million cases of "strep throat" reported each year in the United States. It is caused by the group A streptococcus germ. Many people carry the bacteria in the throat or on the skin and do not have symptoms of disease. The germs usually cause mild infections of the throat resulting in inflammation. However, it may spread to other parts of the body, such as blood or lungs, and cause severe illness that can be fatal.

Transmission and symptoms

The germs are spread by person-to-person contact through nasal or throat discharges. They may also be transmitted through contact with an open wound on the skin. It has not been shown that the bacteria are spread by any means other than person-to-person contact. People who carry the germs and do not have symptoms are much less contagious than people who have symptoms.

The symptoms range from no symptoms to severe symptoms, and in some cases, even death. Mild illnesses include strep throat

(throat swelling and soreness) and impetigo (skin sores). There may also be a slight fever associated with it. Severe disease occurs when the bacteria spread to other parts of the body. This may occur as a result of breaks in the skin that allow the bacteria to enter into the tissues or when a person is immune compromised in some way. This leads to diseases such as necrotizing fasciitis (NF) and streptococcal toxic shock syndrome (STSS). NF causes severe pain and tissue destruction, which can result in amputation. STSS causes severe illness resulting in major organ failure. Death occurs in about 20 percent of NF cases and over half of STSS cases.[1] Strep infection can also trigger an autoimmune reaction in susceptible children, causing rheumatic fever where there is inflammation of the inside of the heart and its valves. Rheumatic fever is the leading cause of heart disease in young children worldwide. Below are warning signs of rheumatic fever. Children experiencing these symptoms after strep infections should be seen by a physician immediately.

- Persistent fevers
- Rashes
- Loss of body control, involuntary movements

Risk groups

Everyone is at risk contracting group A streptococcal infections; however, noninvasive infections occur most often among school-aged children. Severe infections occur most often in specific groups, including elderly people; immune-compromised people; those who have chronic respiratory disease, cardiac disease, or diabetes; and children with chickenpox. Specific ethnic groups at risk for invasive infections include African and Native Americans.

"MONO"

Germs

Another common infection of the throat is infectious mononucleosis. It is caused by the Epstein-Barr virus (EBV), a member of the herpesvirus family. It is one of the most common viruses that infect humans. After a person has been infected with EBV, it is unlikely that he will get sick upon future exposure. By adulthood most people have been exposed to EBV and are no longer at risk of becoming infected. The CDC reports that in the United States as many as 95 percent of adults between the ages of thirty-five and forty have been infected with EBV.[2]

Transmission and symptoms

EBV is transmitted by person-to-person contact. Commonly referred to as the "kissing disease," it is passed from one person to another by close intimate contact via saliva. The virus may be present for up to six weeks before causing symptoms. Therefore people are able to unknowingly spread the virus to others for weeks. It may be transmitted from the saliva of both healthy and sick individuals. Some healthy adults (carriers) may continuously transmit the virus to others.

Risk groups

Infants can become infected at a very young age, but the symptoms are rarely severe. Young children may have very mild symptoms including sore throat and transient fever. Adolescents and young adults are infected at a much greater rate. EBV causes infectious mononucleosis in this group 35–50 percent of the time.[3] The symptoms of infectious mononucleosis include sore throat, swollen lymph glands, and fever. These usually completely resolve within one to two months. Sometimes infections may even involve complications such as swollen liver, spleen, heart problems, and problems with the central nervous system, but these complications are rare. By middle to late adulthood, people who have been previously exposed to EBV do not have symptoms.

EBV has also been shown to remain in the immune system of some people in an inactive state (dormancy). Sometimes the virus can reactivate and is commonly found in the saliva of infected persons. When this occurs, people generally do not have symptoms. Dormant viruses have been found to be associated with two forms of cancer: nasopharygeal carcinoma (upper respiratory tract) and Burkitt's lymphoma (lymph nodes). These are very rare forms of cancer, and the causes are still unknown despite the association with dormant EBV.

PREVENTION OF STREP THROAT AND "MONO"

One reason that group A streptococcus and EBV are so common is because they can spread from people who do not have symptoms.

The EBV can spread for a period of weeks, and some people are lifelong carriers of the virus. This is also the reason that it is almost impossible to prevent both of these infections. Some of the ways to minimize the spread of the disease among people who have symptoms are through isolation and hand washing (strep throat only). However, unless you are willing to completely isolate yourself from everyone indefinitely, there is no true preventive measure to be taken; that is, in the natural realm. Of course, this is not a desirable option. This is a time when the spiritual realm provides the only answer for the prevention of disease. This is truly a time when faith can be applied and when it is necessary to call on the Lord.

> Now faith is the substance of things hoped for,
> the evidence of things not seen.
> —HEBREWS 11:1

Trust Him to take care of you and your family.

LET'S RECAP

Infections of the ears and throat are very common, especially among children. Ear infections occur more frequently in younger children because the ears have not yet completely developed. Usually as children get older, ear infections become less common. It is important to take children to see a health professional if you suspect they have an ear infection. If left untreated, these infections can lead to permanent damage. Throat infections are also very common among children. Both strep throat and infectious mononucleosis can spread from people who do not have symptoms. Therefore, prevention of these two diseases is more difficult. Both of these diseases may also be complicated and lead to more severe infections. If a sore throat is accompanied by a fever, it is important to seek medical attention. Most importantly, seek the Lord in prayer and in faith for the health and well-being of your family.

Now that we have reviewed some common infectious diseases of the respiratory tract, ears, and throat, it is time to move on to diseases that affect other organs.

Chapter 7

DIARRHEA

Have you ever been with a group of people and had a sudden uncontrollable urge to run to the restroom? An even worse situation is to be with that special someone and have to make a mad dash for the closest thing resembling a toilet. These are the times when you wish you had made the quality decision to *stay home*. Probably one of the most uncomfortable illnesses caused by germs is diarrhea. It usually does not last for longer than a few days, but when it's over, boy, are you relieved. (No pun intended!)

This chapter describes diarrhea, a common infection caused by many germs. Both diarrhea and vomiting are direct evidence of infection. They are your body's way of telling you that it will get rid of the germs by any means necessary. If either occurs over a long period of time, they can cause severe pain and result in dehydration, which can be life threatening if not treated promptly.

THE MYTHS

You may recall hearing people say that they contracted the "stomach flu" because they were vomiting and had diarrhea. You may have also heard people say that they contracted "food poisoning" because they were vomiting and had diarrhea after eating at a restaurant. Both are more likely misunderstandings of what has caused infections of the gastrointestinal tract.

THE TRUTH

Actually, there is no such disease as the "stomach flu." The only flu is the disease caused by influenza viruses. Also "food poisoning" can more accurately be described, as an infection by one of the many germs that cause diarrhea, a condition known as gastroenteritis. Gastroenteritis involves the stomach and intestines. There are several groups of viruses, bacteria, and parasites that can cause this condition (Table 2).

TRANSMISSION AND SYMPTOMS

Most germs that cause diarrhea spread via the fecal-to-oral mode of transmission. This means that they were ingested from contaminated food or water. This form of contamination may occur by poor sanitation or hygiene, improper food handing techniques, or improper waste disposal. Often it occurs as a simple failure to wash hands properly. The germs may also be spread by close person-to-person contact; however, this is far less common. Noroviruses are the leading cause of gastroenteritis. In a study conducted by CDC involving outbreaks of diarrhea between 1997 and 2000, a total of 201 (86 percent) of 233 were positive for noroviruses.[1] Fifty-seven percent of the cases were found to be caused by contaminated food, while only 16 percent were caused by person-to-person contact.

Table 2: Common Infectious Agents That Cause Gastroenteritis (Diarrhea)[2]		
VIRUSES	**BACTERIA**	**PARASITES**
Noroviruses	*Escherichia coli*	*Cryptosporidium parvum*
Rotaviruses	*Clostridium difficile*	*Cyclospora cayetanensis*
Adenoviruses	*Campylobacter*	*Entamoeba histolytica*
Astroviruses	*Salmonella enteridis*	*Giardia intestinalis*
Enteroviruses	*Listeria monotogenes*	*Microsporidia*
HIV	*Shigella sp*	*Dientamoeba fragilis*

The symptoms include watery, or even bloody, stool often accompanied by abdominal cramps and pain. Fever may or may not be associated with the diarrhea. Vomiting may also accompany the diarrhea. The symptoms often depend on the age of the infected person. Symptoms usually disappear within one to two weeks, but if they persist for longer periods of time, the condition is referred to as persistent or chronic.

PREVENTION

The chances of getting infected by germs that cause diarrhea can be greatly reduced by applying the methods listed below. Disinfection is the process of killing germs and is usually done by using chlorine bleach or bleach-based cleaners.

To prevent infection with germs that cause diarrhea:
- Wash hands frequently.
- Disinfect contaminated items and surfaces.
- Wash soiled clothing and other articles.
- Avoid food or water that is thought to be contaminated.

GERM TIP #6

These methods of prevention are described in the Book of Leviticus. The scriptures below describe specific instructions for dealing with contaminated surfaces, clothing, and other items.

> And whoever sits on anything on which he who has the discharge has sat shall wash his clothes and bathe himself in water, and be unclean until the evening.
>
> —LEVITICUS 15:6, AMP

Additionally, the Word of God specifically addresses the importance of cooking food properly and warns of eating contaminated food.

> And the flesh that toucheth any unclean thing shall not be eaten; it shall be burnt with fire: and as for the flesh, all that be clean shall eat thereof.
>
> —LEVITICUS 7:19

So, if you go out to dinner and later cannot stay away from the restroom, you should have an idea of what is going on. More than likely you are infected by one of the germs that cause diarrhea rather than food poisoning. Remember, the best way to prevent the spread of germs that cause this disease is by frequent hand washing.

Chapter 8

SEXUALLY TRANSMITTED DISEASES

Shelly was a twenty-year-old junior in college when she found out that she was HIV positive. Up to then, she had been a healthy young woman with a bright future ahead of her. Shelly's boyfriend, Ronald, attended the same university. They had been dating since their freshman year. Ronald was Shelly's first, and she was happy about it. All of the girls on campus liked him, but he *chose* her.

Shelly later found out that she was not the only girl on campus with whom Ronald had been in a relationship. As a result of Ronald's and the other girls' behavior, they suffered the consequences and became infected with HIV.

AIDS is just one of the many sexually transmitted diseases (STDs). Sexual transmission is person-to-person contact through sex. Often there is an exchange of body fluid, which is how the germs are spread. The symptoms of STDs often involve the sex organs (genitalia), and these symptoms may occur immediately or much later. More than twenty-five diseases are transmitted sexually. National estimates are that there are nearly fifteen million new STD cases each year. This chapter includes information about some of the germs that cause common STDs. This topic is important because STDs affect so many young people worldwide. Also, the Bible provides instructions that are foolproof for prevention of STDs.

RISK GROUPS

The Division of STD Prevention at the CDC conducts age-related studies of STDs in the United States. STDs occur most often among adolescents and young adults. This group is at greater risk. For example, in 2003, the rate of chlamydia among women was greater in the group of fifteen- to nineteen-year-olds and twenty- to twenty-four-year-olds than any other age group.[1] Similarly, the rate of gonorrhea among women fifteen to nineteen years old was also greater in 2003.[2] The rate of syphilis has also been reported as much greater among young men and women. In 2003, the rate of syphilis was greatest among women ages twenty to twenty-four and men thirty-five to thirty-nine.[3]

The most common STDs among young people are chlamydia and gonorrhea. Fortunately, because they are caused by bacteria, they can be treated with antibiotics. However, often they can go undetected and result in severe complications, especially in women. This can result in severe complications and increased transmission to other people.

There are many different types of STDs, and they are caused by different types of germs. Below is a brief description of common STDs grouped by the type of germs that cause them.

GERMS

Viruses

- Genital herpes—recurring lesions in genital areas. At this time, there is no cure. Complications affect the nervous system, childbirth, and newborns.
- Cervical dysplasia—abnormal growth of cells on the cervix of the uterus. Complications may lead to cervical cancer.
- AIDS—an infection of immune cells that help fight infection (T cells). At this time, there is no cure. Complications cause people to become susceptible to opportunistic pathogens and are fatal.

Bacteria

- Gonorrhea—inflammation of the reproductive organs. Complications may affect reproductive organs, childbirth, and newborns.
- Chlamydia—inflammation of the reproductive organs. Complications may affect reproductive organs, childbirth, and newborns.
- Syphilis—lesions in the genitalia, rectum, urethra, and mouth. Complications may cause neurological damage, problems during childbirth and with the newborn.

Parasites

- Trichomonas—inflammation of genitalia (usually women). Complications lead to severe abdominal pain.
- Giardiasis—inflammation in gastrointestinal tract, watery or bloody stool (usually homosexual men). Complications may lead to dehydration.
- Amebiasis—inflammation in gastrointestinal tract, watery or bloody stool (usually homosexual men). Complications are rare.
- Scabies—intense itching in infected areas (genitalia). Complications lead to severe lesions.

Fungi

- Vulvovaginitis—inflammation of the vagina and vulva, causing discharge and itching. Complications include recurrent infections and severe discomfort.

PREVENTION

Health-care professionals suggest prophylactics such as condoms to prevent the spread of STDs. However, they are not 100 percent effective. In 2000 the National Institutes of Health (NIH), CDC, and other government agencies evaluated latex condoms and STDs.[4] Their conclusion was that while latex condoms can reduce the risks, condom use *cannot guarantee protection* from any STD. The surest way to prevent STDs is to abstain from sexual relations or to be in a long-term relationship with one person who is known to be uninfected. As in the story of Shelly and Ronald, often STDs are spread between people who have been involved in sexual relations outside of marriage. The Bible clearly instructs us about abstinence from sex outside a monogamous marriage.

> For this is the will of God, even your sanctification, that ye should abstain from fornication.
> —1 THESSALONIANS 4:3

When God gave humankind instruction not to have sex outside of marriage, He did so to protect us physically as well as emotionally.

Chapter 9

DISEASES FROM PETS

For Katie's seventh birthday, her parents bought her an adorable kitten, which she named Buttons. One day while she was playing with Buttons, the kitten scratched her. Katie didn't tell her parents what happened for fear of losing the kitten. A couple of days later, Katie did not feel well enough to go to school. When her mom entered her bedroom to awaken her, Katie told her mom she was tired and did not feel well. Anna, Katie's mom, felt her forehead; she felt warm. She quickly grabbed the thermometer to take Katie's temperature. Her fever was 101° F. When she pulled the covers back and quickly examined Katie's body, she noticed Katie's neck and underarms were swollen. She rushed to get Katie and herself dressed and immediately headed to the doctor's office. Anna tried to remain calm on the outside but was completely terrified on the inside. Questions kept running through her mind: *Was it something she ate? Is somebody in her class sick? Did she catch something from the places we've been in the past few days? The restaurant or mall?*

After they arrived at the doctor's office, Katie's vitals were taken immediately. During this time the nurse began asking a series of questions about things she may have eaten, where she had been, and to whom Katie may have been exposed. Right about the time the nurse completed her questions she noticed something peculiar. There were small scratches on Katie's forearm. Upon careful observation, the nurse observed that the injury appeared a couple of days old and infected. Anna and the nurse asked Katie about the injury. Katie explained that her new kitten, Buttons, had scratched her while they were playing. She did not say anything to her parents because she did not want them to be upset with Buttons. Katie had contracted cat scratch disease, a bacterial infection transmitted to humans from cats. It usually causes mild infection at the point of injury; however, if untreated, the infection can be complicated. Katie was treated with antibiotics.

They're cute and cuddly, and we can't imagine life without them. They are our household pets. Our pets provide companionship, comfort, and unconditional love. Pets provide many benefits to humans; however, many can also transmit diseases. Diseases transmitted from animals to humans are called *zoonoses*. This chapter will provide some information about common zoonoses passed from household pets and other animals. Of course, not all of the diseases are described here, but some of the common diseases are briefly described. My purpose is not to make pet owners fearful or to discourage people from buying pets, but to provide information to help keep both you and your pets healthy. Pets are wonderful and can provide great health benefits.

VIRAL DISEASES: RABIES

Rabies is caused by the rabies virus. People usually get rabies from the bite of infected wild animals such as foxes, raccoons, and skunks, but domestic animals such as cats and dogs may also transmit it. It may take from weeks to years for people to show symptoms of rabies. Early symptoms include headache and fever. What follows are symptoms associated with the nervous system such as confusion and mood swings; the disease is usually fatal when the symptoms progress to this point. Rabies can be prevented in domestic animals by keeping animals vaccinated and under close supervision when around other pets. The best way to prevent rabies from wild animals is to avoid direct contact with them.

BACTERIAL DISEASES

Campylobacter infections

Many germs can be transmitted in more than one way. *Camplylobacter sp* can cause bacterial infection. Sometimes humans can get infected from the stool of an infected animal such as a dog or cat. It causes mild to severe infections of the gastrointestinal tract, including diarrhea and abdominal cramps often accompanied by fever. A rare complication is a disease of the nervous system. The best way to prevent *Campylobacter* infections is to wash hands after coming into contact with animal stool.

Cat scratch disease

As you read in the anecdote at the beginning of this chapter, cat scratch disease (CSD) is transmitted to humans from the bite or scratch of an infected cat. CSD is caused by the bacteria *Bartonella henselae*. Infection usually occurs at the site of injury. The CDC reports that about 40 percent of cats carry the bacteria at some point in their lifetime. Symptoms you may experience include fever, headache, loss of appetite, and swollen lymph nodes. The best ways to prevent CSD are to avoid cat bites and scratches. Avoid rough-housing with a cat, especially a kitten. If you are injured by a cat, wash the site of injury immediately and do not allow the cat to lick your open wounds.

Hemolytic uremic syndrome

As of this writing, there was an outbreak of hemolytic uremic syndrome (HUS) in Florida. *Escherichia coli* bacteria can cause HUS. As with most germs, you can become infected in more than one way. The *E. coli* bacteria can be found in contaminated food such as meat or milk products, but it can also be found in animal secretions and waste. Traveling petting zoos were believed to be the source for the Florida outbreak.

I would suggest that parents not use the media as the source of information for infectious diseases. If there has been an outbreak, then check your local or state health department for specific information. As a rule, I would tell parents not to exclude their children from educational field trips because of a media scare.

Most established petting zoos and farms that are open to the public should be required to have inspections and meet health codes to ensure that the animals are healthy. If the zoo or farm doesn't practice health department guidelines, then don't participate. I would suggest that parents review general healthy habits with their children:

1. Do not come in contact with animal secretions— saliva, nasal secretions and, especially, waste. If so, wash your hands immediately and thoroughly.
2. Wash hands after visiting the farm and, more importantly, before eating.

3. Never allow children to put their hands or objects (such as a pacifier or a cup) into their mouths after petting an animal.

Leptosporosis

Leptosporosis is a disease caused by the bacteria called *leptospires.* The bacteria can cause disease in humans and domestic animals and has been reported worldwide. The bacteria are spread through the urine of infected animals and can enter humans through the skin or mucous membranes. The symptoms in humans are usually flu-like, but sometimes severe infections of the kidneys, lungs, brain, and heart are observed. Often pets do not have symptoms. The best prevention of the disease is to wash areas that have been in contact with pets.

Salmonellosis

This disease is caused by many different types of *Salmonella* bacteria. The bacteria may cause infection in humans and many kinds of animals, including dogs, cats, birds, horses, and reptiles. Humans get it most often from eating contaminated food, but infected animals can pass it on in their stool. Symptoms of salmonellosis include diarrhea, fever, and stomach pain and usually last for about one week. If the infection is spread, it must be treated with antibiotics. Washing your hands before eating, especially when in contact with animal waste, may help prevent it.

Yersiniosis

Yersiniosis is caused by the bacteria *Yersinia enterocolitica.* Humans usually contract the disease from contact with infected pigs, but it may be transmitted from other animals including dogs, cats, rabbits, and horses. It may be passed from the stool of an infected animal. Symptoms include fever, stomach pain, and diarrhea and can last from one to three weeks. Severity of the symptoms is dependent upon the person's age. Children have symptoms more often than adults. Washing your hands after coming into contact with animal waste, not eating undercooked meats, and drinking only pasteurized milk products may prevent it.

PARASITIC DISEASES

Hookworms

Many different types of parasites cause hookworm infections. Young animals such as puppies and kittens are very likely to be infected with hookworms. These infections may be complicated because of the complex life cycle of the parasites. Infected animals pass the eggs in their stool, and the eggs hatch and develop into larvae, which may survive in soil and dirt. The eggs and larvae may enter the body through contaminated dirt or soil. They may migrate through the skin, causing skin infections, or if ingested, they may cause infections in the intestines. The best ways to prevent hookworm infections are to have pets dewormed and to avoid walking barefoot in soil and dirt.

Roundworms

Roundworm infections are caused by the *Toxacara* group of parasites. In the United States an estimated ten thousand cases occur annually. As with hookworms, infected animals, such as dogs and cats, pass on the eggs through their stool. The eggs are transmitted to humans by ingestion from soil or other contaminated surfaces. Two forms of infection generally occur: infection of the eye or the nervous system. Most infections in humans are very mild; however, the more severe cases often occur in children. The best ways to prevent roundworm infections are to have pets treated for worms, clean their areas, and encourage children to wash their hands after playing in dirt and soil.

Tapeworms

Dipylidium is the most common tapeworm of dogs and cats in the United States. It is transmitted to pets when they ingest an infected flea. Once ingested, the larvae develop into adults inside the animal. Adult tapeworms are made of segments called proglottids that break and pass in the stool of an infected animal. The proglottids are hard and may stick to the anal area of pets after they pass stool. Infection in humans is most common among children and occurs when children ingest infected fleas. An infected child may have proglottids around the anal area after having a bowel movement. Treatment for tapeworms is either oral ingestion or an injection of an antiparasitic drug that dissolves the tapeworms in the intestines. The best ways to prevent tapeworm infections is to have pets treated for fleas and worms. Also, cleaning up their waste promptly and immediately washing hands will help to prevent tapeworm infections. Don't allow children to play in areas soiled with pet waste, and always have children wash their hands after playing with pets.

FUNGAL DISEASES

Ringworm

Ringworms are skin and scalp infections caused by a variety of fungi. The fungus is transmitted to humans by direct contact with an infected animal. Many animals may transmit ringworms, including dogs, cats, horses, and farm animals. Scalp infections usually result in a patch of scaly skin with some hair loss. Skin infections cause ring-shaped rashes that are also scaly and may be red and itchy. The best way to prevent ringworm infections from animals is to wash hands after direct contact with pets.

GERM TIP #7

To prevent the spread of infectious diseases from pets:
- Keep vaccinations up to date for all dogs, cats, and other pets.
- Control fleas on your pets and in their environment (indoor and outdoor).
- Encourage each family member to wash their hands after playing with pets and after playing outdoors.
- Immediately clean any scratches or wounds that result from playing with pets.
- Always clean up after your pets.
- Do not allow children to play in areas where there is animal waste.
- Avoid stray animals, and ensure that your pets do not come into contact with them.

Pets can be wonderful additions to any household. If pets are properly cared for, they can offer great health benefits to the entire family. Continue to follow the preventive measures I have outlined for you, and reduce the risks of pet-related germs.

UNIT 3

GERMS AND CHRONIC DISEASES

Chapter 10

CANCER

Most of us know someone that has suffered from cancer. My mother became very ill and was diagnosed with a rare form of cancer of the urethra. After undergoing surgery, she quickly adjusted to her new life. A couple of months later, we were informed that the cancer had spread to other parts of her body. Even as she underwent chemotherapy, my mother maintained a good attitude. Unfortunately, the chemotherapy did not work, and she passed away in 2001. Not once did she complain about her condition.

Like me, many of you have lost family members and friends to the disease. This chapter will describe several different forms of cancer that have been linked to infectious agents. Evidently, germs appear to be more important than what people originally thought. Not only are they responsible for many infectious diseases, they are also linked to several different forms of cancer. There is so much that people don't know about cancer, so I will begin with the basics.

WHAT IS CANCER?

There are millions of people in the United States who are living with it today. Cancer is the second leading cause of death in the United States. Over one million people get it each year. It is estimated that in the United States one-half of all men and one-third of all women will develop it in their lifetimes. The CDC's National Center for Health Statistics reports that compared to the rate in 1950, the cancer rate was 0.2 percent higher in 2001, while the rates for other chronic diseases decreased during this time.[1]

God designed our bodies so that all functions for growth and development occur in an orderly fashion. For example, normal cells in our bodies grow and divide in an orderly fashion. When we are young, they grow and divide very rapidly, but when we become adults, they generally grow and divide more slowly, usually only to replace dead or dying cells or to repair injuries. Cancer develops when cells *do not* grow in an orderly fashion. It is a general term used for diseases that are characterized by abnormal and uncontrolled cell growth. The resulting abnormal cells can clump together and form a tumor, which can invade and destroy normal tissues. Cancer cells from the tumor can spread through the bloodstream and lymph system, forming new tumors in other parts of the body.

Not all tumors are cancerous. Some tumors are benign, meaning they do not spread to other parts of the body and are usually not life threatening. Malignant tumors can spread and cause serious diseases.

History

There are descriptions of cancer recorded throughout history. The first documented cases are believed to have occurred in Egypt at approximately 1600 B.C. The descriptions are of breast tumors, and it was recorded that there were no treatments. The name *cancer* is derived from the terms *carcinos* and *carcinoma*, credited to the Greek physician Hippocrates, who used these terms to describe tumors. From the fifteenth to seventeenth century, scientists began to apply the scientific method to study the human body and disease. The first autopsies were performed, which enabled scientists to understand things such as blood flow and circulation. Most importantly, it enabled them to relate the illnesses of patients to the cause after death. These findings led to the study of cancer.

Probably one of the biggest contributions to the study of cancer was the invention of the microscope. During the nineteenth century Rudolf Virchow was able to use the microscope to observe the effects of cancer at a microscopic level. This provided doctors with much more insight to the effects of cancer. It also enabled doctors to carefully observe tumors and led to operations for surgical removal of tumors.

WHAT ARE THE DIFFERENT TYPES OF CANCER?

There have been more than one hundred forms of cancer identified. It has been observed in every major tissue and organ of the body, including the brain, bone, skin, soft tissues, and blood. There are forms of cancer that primarily affect children. However, 77 percent of cases occur in people that are age fifty-five and older.[2] It may affect all types of people but differences are observed among different ethnic groups.

WHAT CAUSES CANCER?

Cancer is caused by damaged DNA. DNA is the material that contains the genetic information for an individual and is found in all cells. Our body is a remarkable machine that is able to repair most forms of damage that occurs, including damage to DNA. In cancerous cells the DNA no longer undergoes repair at a normal rate; therefore, the cells do not grow and divide normally. Sometimes people can inherit damaged DNA from their parents. This accounts for the genetic or inherited forms of cancer. DNA can also be damaged by exposure to things in the environment.

Risk factors

There are some risk factors that cannot be avoided. One example is genetics. As mentioned previously, some people inherit damaged DNA from their parents. Also, a person is more likely to get cancer at some point in their life if it is a part of their family's medical history. This does not mean that they *will* develop cancer; the risk is just greater. Another unavoidable risk factor is age. As we get older, unfortunately our risk of getting cancer increases. Gender and ethnicity also contribute to a person's risk. According to the American Cancer Society, Caucasian and African American males have the highest rate of cancer deaths more than any other race.[3]

Several habits that have been linked to cancer can be avoided. Probably the best example of a habit to avoid is smoking and use of tobacco. While it is important to mention that although not everyone who smokes gets cancer, smoking does increase the risks. Smoking has been linked to cancers of the lung, throat, mouth, esophagus, bladder, kidneys, and other organs. Drinking alcohol has also been shown to increase the risk of cancers of the mouth, throat, and other organs. Risks are believed to be especially high for people who drink and smoke. Other environmental factors such as radiation have been shown to cause cancer. Exposure to excess sunlight without protection has been associated with skin cancer. Many chemicals and other substances such as benzene, arsenic, hydrocarbons, and asbestos have also been shown to cause cancer. It is estimated that environmental factors such as tobacco use, chemicals, radiation, diet, and infectious diseases cause about 75 percent of cancer cases in the United States.[4]

GERMS AND CANCER

As early as the nineteenth century, it was believed that infectious agents can cause different forms of cancer. A great deal of research efforts were directed toward finding germs that cause cancers, unsuccessfully. With the advancements in biotechnology, research in this area has been very successful. Several forms of cancer have now been linked to infectious agents. The remainder of this chapter will describe some forms of cancer that have been associated with infectious agents. It is important to mention that the infectious agents are not necessarily the only cause of these cancers.

Cervical cancer

The uterus, a reproductive organ in women, has two parts: the upper part called the body, which holds the developing baby, and the lower part called the cervix, which connects the body to the vagina. Cancer of the cervix takes some time to develop. It begins at the lining of the cervix when the cervical cells change form, a condition known as dysplasia. Cervical dysplasia can be detected early with a Pap smear test and treated before the cells become cancerous. This is why it is recommended that women have them routinely (every two to three years depending on age and history or every year for women who are sexually active). Sometimes this condition disappears without treatment, but most often treatment is required to prevent cancer. The cause of cervical dysplasia is infection with human papillomavirus. The virus is transmitted during sexual intercourse. This is the only mode of transmission as it related to cervical cancer. It must be mentioned that this virus has also been associated with warts when it is transmitted differently. To date the only effective cure is surgical and only if detected early.

Clinical trials for a vaccine for human papillomavirus are currently underway. If successful, this will be one of the first vaccines to prevent a form of cancer caused by an infectious agent.

Kaposi's sarcoma

Sarcomas are cancers that develop in connective tissues such as blood, bone, muscle, cartilage, and fat. Kaposi's sarcoma (KS) was named after the late Dr. Moritz Kaposi, who described the disease in the late 1800s. There are several different types of KS, each differing in the symptoms and organs affected. KS causes tumors to develop in the tissue beneath the skin or mucous membranes. Often it appears as raised patches called lesions. These lesions may be very painful and can cause disfigurement, but they are usually not fatal. In most cases they cause no symptoms. Other symptoms associated with KS include pain and swelling of the appendages. KS is caused by the Kaposi sarcoma-associated herpesvirus (KSHV). For years KS was a rare disease; however, in recent years it has been associated with AIDS. Treatment for KS often includes surgery, radiation therapy, and chemotherapy.

Liver cancer

The liver performs several different functions that are necessary for our survival. It secretes bile into the intestines to help with digestion and absorption of fats. It processes and stores nutrients absorbed from the intestines. It is involved in the removal of toxins and waste from the body. It also produces blood-clotting factors and the cholesterol needed to make bile salts. The liver is made up of several different types of cells, which is why it is possible for different types of tumors to form there. Hepatitis B virus can chronically infect cells of the liver called hepatocytes. The virus is spread from blood or body fluids from an infected person. Having unprotected sex or sharing a needle with an infected person are examples of how the virus may be spread. In approximately 6 percent of the people infected after age five, the virus will not be cleared, and they will experience chronic liver damage.[5] Fifteen to 25 percent of these people die from cirrhosis of the liver or liver cancer.[6] Treatments can be performed if tumors develop and are diagnosed early. Treatments of liver cancer are surgery, radiation therapy, and chemotherapy.

Nasopharyngeal cancer

The nasopharynx is a chamber in the back of the nose at the base of the skull. It is located directly in back of the entrance into the nasal passage. It is lined with several layers of tissue containing many different types of cells. Several different types of tumors can develop in this area, and unfortunately the tumors cause severe disease by the time they are diagnosed. Several different types of cancers can develop, but nasopharyngeal carcinoma (NPC) is the most common malignant tumor of the nasopharynx. Infection with Epstein-Barr virus (EBV) and the herpes virus that cause infectious mononucleosis has been linked to NPC, although infection alone is not believed to be the cause of NPC. The treatments for NPC are radiation therapy, chemotherapy, and occasionally surgery.

Summary of germs and different forms of cancer

To summarize, there are several forms of cancer that are now known to be associated with infectious agents. Cervical cancer is caused by the human papillomavirus and is transmitted through sexual intercourse. Early detection through routine Pap smears is the key to preventing this form of cancer. Kaposi's sarcoma is a form of cancer that affects the tissues and mucous membranes. It most commonly affects people that have been infected with HIV, although HIV is not believed to be the cause of the disease. It is thought to be more prevalent among people suffering from AIDS because they have weak immune systems. Liver cancer has been shown to be associated with the hepatitis B virus, but this is not the only cause.

PREVENTION

As mentioned previously, several risk factors of cancer cannot be avoided, but others can. Your lifestyle can have a big effect on your risk of developing cancer. A large percentage of the cases of cancer are caused by environmental factors. Therefore, several lifestyle decisions can instantly reduce your risk of developing the disease.

The first lifestyle change that a person can make to reduce the risk of developing cancer is to quit smoking, if he/she is a smoker. Smoking causes damage to nearly all of the organs in the body and has been linked to several different types of cancer. I know that it is easier said than done by a nonsmoker, but the truth is that I *was* a smoker for years. Smoking is an addiction. I am fully aware of how difficult it may be for some people to stop smoking. I made several unsuccessful attempts to quit over the years. I remember how frustrated I used to get when I heard nonsmokers tell people to quit. Finally, I realized that I could not do it on my own, and I prayed. It was not until I made the decision to change in my heart and realized that I could not do it on my own that I received the victory. I thank God for deliverance from the addiction. Today there are nonprescription and prescription drugs and support groups to help people quit smoking. Quitting smoking is one of the best things that you can do for yourself and your family.

If you have not already, the second lifestyle change that you can make is to eat right. Eating healthy meals will not only decrease the risk of cancer but will also improve your overall health. Choose to exchange fresh fruits and vegetables for fried foods in your diet. Stay away from processed foods and foods that are high in either saturated or trans fats. Also, if you are overweight, decrease your food intake to reach and maintain an optimal body weight.

One simple way to decrease your food intake is the 2PD Omer Approach.[7] This is a simple diet based upon the only principle that has proven to work for permanent weight loss—eating less. The 2PD Omer Approach is to decrease your food intake to a total of two pounds of food each day. This, of course, would mean that you must purchase a food scale and weigh your food each day. This amount of food is sufficient to sustain everyone—big, small, short, tall, old, or young. It is also based on biblical principles. In Exodus 16:16, the Lord commanded that His people each eat just one *omer* (Hebrew word that means "a certain weight") of *manna* (food), which He provided every morning except on the Sabbath mornings for the forty years His people wandered in the desert. This amount was the same for each person regardless of age, size, gender, or activity and proved to be all that a person needed, because no one died from starvation during the forty years in the desert. This "one size fits all" concept is hard for many to believe, but it is the basis for the 2PD Approach.

Another way to decrease the risk of cancer is to exercise. This does not mean that a person has to spend hours in the gym each day to remain healthy. Find a form of exercise that works well for you and stick with it. Walking, bike riding, skating, jogging, dancing, and playing sports are all examples. The important thing is to find something that you enjoy and stick with it.

Many other environmental risk factors for cancer can be reduced fairly easily. Decreasing prolonged exposure to the sun will decrease the risk of certain forms of skin cancer. Also the use of ultraviolet radiation (UV) protection sunscreen and sunglasses may help. Many of the chemical exposure risk factors are no longer a problem in the United States because the government has set occupational guidelines and standards to decrease public exposure to carcinogenic chemicals. Also, the amount of radiation that is used routinely by doctors and dentists is not hazardous.

LET'S RECAP

In summary, cancer is uncontrolled cell growth. It occurs as a result of damaged DNA. People can inherit damaged DNA from their parents, or DNA may become damaged from environmental factors. Also, some forms of cancers have been shown to be caused by or associated with infections with germs. Two ways to prevent the risk of cancer is to choose to avoid unsafe behaviors, such as smoking, and maintaining a healthy lifestyle. Both are quality choices that are well worth the overall health benefits.

Chapter 11

ACQUIRED IMMUNODEFICIENCY
SYNDROME (AIDS)

One of the most devastating chronic diseases linked to an infectious agent is AIDS. When AIDS was first reported in the United States in 1981,[1] we knew very little about this deadly disease. What we once thought to be linked to homosexuality now affected everyone regardless of their sexuality. We now know that mothers who are carriers of HIV can pass it on to their unborn children during birth and after birth through breastfeeding. Drug abusers sharing needles can transmit it through contaminated needles. Before we knew the severity of this chronic disease, blood banks unknowingly collected contaminated blood from blood donors with AIDS, and eventually that contaminated blood would infect healthy, innocent people. Since then, however, blood banks carefully screen each donor for HIV and other transmittable diseases, such as hepatitis B.

AIDS is caused by the human immunodeficiency virus (HIV), a retrovirus. Since 1981, more than nine hundred thousand cases of AIDS have been reported in the United States.[2]

Although there are several ways that HIV can be spread, the most common mode of transmission is direct contact (person-to-person, sexual). The virus can enter the body through the vagina, penis, rectum, and mouth.

WHAT IS AIDS?

HIV infects and kills the body's T cells, which are cells that play an important role in our body's specific immunity. (See chapter 2.) Many people who become infected with HIV do not have symptoms right away, while some may develop transient flu-like symptoms. Over time the virus continues to infect and kill T cells. The fewer the number of T cells, the less capable the body is of mounting a specific immune response against infectious agents. This makes the body vulnerable to infections by germs that our body would normally be able to fight off, especially opportunistic pathogens. Eventually the number of T cells remaining becomes too low to fight off the infections that normally do not affect healthy people. AIDS is the name given to advanced stages of HIV infection. It occurs when an HIV-infected person's T cell count is very low compared to that in a healthy person.

Opportunistic infections

Opportunistic infections from bacteria, viruses, fungi, and parasites become severe in people who have developed AIDS. Many of the infectious diseases described in previous chapters become more common, including diarrhea, pneumonia, and cancers such as Kaposi's sarcoma. Some of the symptoms associated with the opportunistic infections among people with AIDS are fever, weight loss, vision loss, nausea, vomiting, coughing, and shortness of breath. Neurological symptoms such as forgetfulness are also observed.

Risk groups

Since HIV can be transmitted in a variety of ways, people with certain behaviors are at a greater risk of becoming infected. Included among risk groups are people who have unprotected sex with an infected person, people who have unprotected sex with a person whose HIV status is not known, and intravenous drug users that share needles.

Detection

As mentioned previously, some people do not get symptoms immediately after infection with HIV. It is therefore important for people who are at risk to be tested. HIV infection is diagnosed by tests that identify antibodies to the virus. It may take from three to six months for these antibodies to become detectable. For this reason, it is best to be tested three to twelve months after exposure. The surest way to be certain one is HIV free is to be tested, discontinue risky behaviors, and then be tested again three to six months later. After providing a blood sample, it usually takes a few days up to a week to get the test results.

Treatments

To date there is no cure for AIDS. However, the FDA has approved several treatments for the disease and the opportunistic infections. One group of drugs is called nucleoside analogs. These drugs prevent processes involved with the virus making copies of itself. One example is AZT, a drug commonly prescribed to AIDS patients. Treatment with this drug delays the spread of HIV to cells in the body. It has also been very effective in preventing the spread of HIV from mother to child during childbirth. Another group of drugs used for the treatment of AIDS is protease inhibitors. These drugs inhibit the activity of some viral proteins. At least six different protease inhibitors have been approved by the FDA for the treatment of AIDS. HIV can easily become resistant to these drugs, so it is often necessary for doctors to prescribe a combination of drugs for effective treatment. This "cocktail" treatment is believed to have significantly reduced the number of AIDS-related deaths.

Prevention

The best way to prevent HIV infection is to refrain from any of the risky behaviors described in this chapter. The CDC recommends that people should either abstain from having sex or protect themselves by using latex condoms. People should not use needles that other people have used. Pregnant women who have become infected with HIV should take AZT during the pregnancy and during labor to reduce the risk of transmitting it to their babies. Importantly, if you are planning to marry, it is recommended that both you and your mate be tested prior to marriage.

DEBUNKING THE MYTHS ABOUT AIDS

Before going further, I would like to clarify some of the misconceptions about transmission of HIV.

HIV is *not* transmitted in the following ways:

- From the environment
- Touching, such as hand shaking and hugs
- Casual kissing
- Saliva, tears, and sweat
- Insect bites

There is no evidence to support that HIV is spread through any of the ways listed above. Research scientists have conducted studies and concluded that HIV does not survive well in the environment. This finding decreases the risks of transmission through the environment and touching. There is also no risk associated with kissing (closed mouth). Even the risk of transmission through open mouth kissing is very low. HIV has been found in the saliva and tears of infected persons, but in very low quantities. There is no evidence that the virus can be transmitted from the saliva, tears, or sweat of an infected person. Although the virus may be found in these body fluids, it is not present in large amounts as in transmission through nursing (drinking large volumes), birth canal (placenta with large amounts of fluid), or in close sexual contact.

Finally, the CDC and other groups have conducted several studies to investigate the transmission of HIV in insects. They have found three factors that decrease this possibility. First, HIV only lives for a short while in insects. Second, insects do not become infected and therefore cannot transmit the virus. Third, biting insects do not travel from one person to next immediately, but rather take the time to digest their meals first.

BIBLICAL PREVENTION

Since sexual contact is the most common mode of transmission for HIV, the best way to prevent infection is to abstain from sex. As discussed in chapter eight, God's plan for our bodies involves sex in a monogamous marriage. First Corinthians 6:18 says that to commit fornication is to sin against our bodies. If we and our partner are obedient to biblical instruction, then we are protected. Isn't it wonderful how God's plan involves protection?

Chapter 12

DISEASES OF MAJOR ORGANS AND TISSUES

When people think about major diseases such as heart disease or diabetes, they usually do not associate such diseases with germs. The truth is that many infectious diseases do not have severe lifelong effects, especially if treated properly. But did you know that many germs have now been associated with chronic diseases as well?

The first investigations of infectious agents being associated with chronic diseases began in the nineteenth century with cancer research. In the years following, scientists tried to find infectious agents as a cause for tumors. After many unsuccessful attempts, the idea became very unpopular. However, recently, increasing amounts of evidence linking chronic diseases to infectious agents are being uncovered. This chapter will describe four chronic diseases that have been associated with infectious agents.

ATHEROSCLEROSIS (HEART DISEASE)

During the time of writing this book I suffered the loss of a dear relative. He died while sleeping. The cause of death was a heart attack, not a very uncommon one. We all know of someone that has suffered from a heart attack. There are several conditions that can lead to a heart attack. One is atherosclerosis. Atherosclerosis is a condition of clogging, narrowing, and hardening of the body's arteries. It occurs when fatty deposits build on the inner walls of arteries and interfere with blood flow. Atherosclerosis is a major component of cardiovascular disease (CVD), which accounts for 29 percent of deaths worldwide.[1] It is estimated that atherosclerosis is the cause of 42 percent of deaths in the United States annually, and it is a major contributor of coronary heart disease.[2]

Recently, there has been much evidence linking atherosclerosis to infectious agents. First, patients with atherosclerosis often have lesions that are very similar to those caused by infectious agents. Second, there has been evidence linking infection with the bacteria *Chlamydia pneumoniae* with atherosclerosis. Several groups have reported an association between infection with the bacteria and the disease.[3] Animal studies have also supported this link.[4] The best evidence is the detection of bacterial components (parts and components) inside lesions from patients with the disease.[5] One would think that if the disease is indeed associated with a bacterial infection, then antibiotics should be a likely treatment. Unfortunately, the use of even powerful antibiotics has not prevented atherosclerotic lesions. This leads professionals to believe that the bacteria are associated with the disease, but may not be the only factor.

DIABETES MELLITUS TYPE 1

Type 1 diabetes, often referred to as juvenile, or insulin-dependent, diabetes, is a chronic disease that occurs when cells of the pancreas produce too little insulin. This form of diabetes normally affects people under the age of thirty, hence the name juvenile. Insulin is a hormone that is required for glucose (sugar) to enter the cells of the body. When there is not enough insulin produced, glucose builds up in the bloodstream and cannot be used for energy by the cells. This is why people who have this form of diabetes require insulin injections. It reduces blood sugar levels by allowing glucose to enter the cells. Symptoms include increased urination and thirst as a result of high blood sugar levels. The CDC conducts surveillance of diabetes (both type 1 and 2) and reports that since 1980, the number of cases of both in the United States has doubled from six to twelve million.[6] Type 1 diabetes represents less than 10 percent of the total cases of diabetes, so most of the increase is coming from type 2 diabetes.

There have been several reports linking type 1 diabetes to infection with a group of viruses called enteroviruses. In studies involving patients with type 1 diabetes, enteroviruses were often detected. Enteroviruses have also been shown to cause diabetes when tested in animals. Also, in a study conducted in Japan, enteroviruses were detected from 37.7 percent of samples collected from children with type 1 diabetes.[7] The investigators concluded that there is an association between type 1 diabetes and enteroviruses.

LYME ARTHRITIS

Many may not think of arthritis as a chronic disease. However, it fits the definition: many patients require long-term care, and the effects are often irreversible. Lyme arthritis is a chronic disease that is known to be caused by germs. It occurs as a late symptom associated with Lyme disease. Lyme disease is caused by the bacteria *Borrelia burgdorferi*. It is transmitted to humans through tick bites and is the most common vector-borne disease in the United States. Early, midterm, and late stages of symptoms are associated with the disease.

Here are some of the early warning signs of Lyme disease:

- Fever and chills
- Headache
- Stiff neck
- Flu-like symptoms
- Fatigue

Lyme disease can be treated with antibiotics. Arthritis occurs in up to 60 percent of untreated patients.[8] Arthritic attacks may occur from several weeks to months. In some patients the arthritis disappears over time; however, about 10 percent are left with irreversibly damaged joints.[9]

PEPTIC ULCERS

Ulcers are another chronic disease because they often recur, cause severe damage to the organs they affect, and require long-term care. A peptic ulcer is a sore or hole on the lining of the stomach or a part of the small intestine called the duodenum. Peptic ulcers can affect people of all ages. The CDC reports that over twenty-five million Americans will suffer from a peptic ulcer at some point during their lifetime.[10] Although stress may contribute to an ulcer, the majority of ulcers are caused by the bacteria *Helicobacter pylori*. *H. pylori* is a bacterium that is found in the gastric mucous membrane or lining of the stomach. When this bacterium erodes the lining of the stomach, sometimes ulcers recur, causing great pain and discomfort to the individual. Antibiotic therapies have been shown to be very effective and can significantly reduce the rate of recurrence among patients.

PREVENTION FOR CHRONIC DISEASES

Many of the risk factors for heart disease and other chronic diseases are the same as those mentioned for cancer. Therefore, prevention is also the same. Examples are eating in moderation and exercising. They are by far the best contributors to overall good health, which can greatly reduce the risk of all chronic diseases. Some germs may be prevented, while for others it is not so clear. For example, the germ that causes Lyme disease may be prevented by dressing properly (fully clothed) when in wooded areas and wearing effective repellants. However, infection by the germs associated with atherosclerosis and ulcers do not have specific preventions. So to maintain overall good health the best advice is to get routine checkups and examinations. Most chronic diseases have a far better chance for successful treatment when they are detected early. A final contributor to good health is the proper attitude. Do not allow the statistics and information to cause you to develop fear. Living in fear may have devastating effects on both your physical and mental health. The Bible describes the effects of fear and tells us that God removes this burden.

> There is no fear in love; but perfect love casteth out fear: because fear hath torment. He that feareth is not made perfect in love.
>
> —1 JOHN 4:18

Allow wisdom and common sense to reign in your life instead of fear. For all of these diseases, the risks can be greatly reduced by doing things that contribute to good health, including healthy eating habits and exercise. Importantly, routine checkups by a doctor greatly increase the chances of successful treatments for all chronic diseases.

UNIT 4

GERM STOPPERS—FIGHTING BACK

Chapter 13

PREVENTION VS. TREATMENT

Jenna did not feel well. It started with a slight fever and scratchy throat. Within a day or two, she had developed a rash and swollen lymph glands in her neck, followed by body aches. The symptoms became so painful and severe that she was rushed to the hospital. The eyes of the emergency room attendant widened when he saw the swelling and hives. He was afraid that the swelling would block Jenna's air passages, making her unable to breathe. There was no waiting involved; Jenna was immediately seen by a physician. She was given an injection of antibiotics and told to remain in bed for the remainder of the week. It took about a week for the swelling and other symptoms to completely disappear.

Jenna had strep throat. The infection had been complicated by an allergic reaction. This is just one of the many complications that can occur as a result of an infection. If Jenna had not been seen right away, the infection could have been fatal. After questioning by the physician, it was found that she had contracted it from her ten-year-old daughter, who, by the way, was not as severely affected. Her daughter had been complaining of a sore throat the week before. Jenna gave her cough medicine, throat lozenges, and pain reliever. Her symptoms were gone by the end of the week. In addition to the medicine, Jenna gave her daughter lots of TLC—hugs and kisses to comfort her during her illness. One night, Jenna even lay in the bed with her daughter to console her. She thought there could be no real harm in this. After all, it was just a sore throat.

We can never be sure of how the symptoms associated with an infection will affect us. Jenna's daughter suffered from a mere sore throat, while Jenna's symptoms were nearly fatal. The antibiotic injection given by the physician is an example of a treatment. There are, however, some things that Jenna could have done differently to avoid contracting the infection. Decreasing the amount of close contact (hugs and kisses) would have decreased the risk of infection. Frequent hand washing during this time may have also decreased the risk of infection. These practices are examples of prevention. They are not foolproof, but they do decrease the risk of infection. Of course, I am not suggesting that you should not show love to family members when they are ill. It is probably just wise to employ some preventive measures while you do so.

PREVENTION OF INFECTIOUS DISEASES: VACCINATION

One way to prevent the spread of infectious diseases is through vaccines. Vaccines are administered orally, by injection, and more recently, by inhalation. They are strongly recommended and should be administered according to the prescribed schedules to prevent unnecessary infections. With the advancements in vaccine development, it is important to be sure that you are aware of the current schedules. If you are unaware of the current recommended immunization schedule, it is important to check with a physician or your local county or state health department. The CDC's National Immunization Program generates a schedule that includes the most recent updates (Table 3).

What are vaccines?

Vaccines take advantage of our body's specific immunity. Remember that specific immunity is our body's ability to recall germs it has been in contact with. Once our body becomes infected with a germ, it can mount a specific immune response against it. We may become ill the first time, but upon subsequent exposures to the same germ our body is able to respond more quickly because it "remembers" the germ. Usually, healthy people do not become ill when infected by the same germs at subsequent times in their lives. Essentially we have become resistant or *immune* to those germs.

This is the driving force behind vaccine development. A vaccine is a low or noninfectious dose of a germ that is given to provide protection by triggering a specific immune response. Often the initial immune response induced by a vaccine is not sufficient to fight an infection with the real germ. This is why for some germs a second or even third dose (booster) is required to be effective. Vaccines are most effective when most of the people in the community have been vaccinated. This prevents the risk of exposure to vaccine-preventable diseases.

The myths

The media has done an effective job of scaring most parents about the dangers of childhood vaccinations, but I am going to debunk some of those myths. It is important for me to address a few of them so that parents will make informed decisions about having their children immunized. Here are three of the common misconceptions about vaccines.

1. Vaccines can cause severe side effects, disease, and can even lead to death.
2. Most people who get diseases have already been vaccinated.
3. The incidence of disease has decreased due to improvements in sanitation, not vaccines.

The truth

Vaccines are actually quite safe, and the side effects are usually very mild. Some examples are a low-grade fever or sniffles for a day or two, which are, of course, preferable to the actual disease symptoms. Vaccines that are given to children routinely have been shown to be effective in 85 to 95 percent of the children that receive them.[1] Some vaccines, such as measles, have an even greater efficacy rate. Finally, the CDC reports that the significant decrease in the number of cases of illnesses in the United States corresponds with introduction of vaccine use.[2]

The history

Today most people in the United States have not seen the effects of diseases such as diphtheria, whooping cough, or rubella. Many young people have not even heard of these diseases. However, in the nineteenth and early twentieth centuries these diseases were very common in the United States, affecting tens of thousands of people and killing many. Many of the diseases that were very common in the United States and many other countries are hardly ever heard of today because of the advancements in vaccine development.

AGE	VACCINE							
mos.-yrs.	*HepB*	*DTaP*	*Hib*	*IPV*	*PCV*	*Influenza*	*MMR*	*Varicella*
0-2 mos.	X							
1-4 mos.	X							
2 mos.		X	X	X	X			
4 mos.		X	X	X	X			
6 mos.		X	X		X			
6-18 mos.	X			X				
6-23 mos.						X		
12-15 mos.			X		X		X	X
15-18 mos.		X						
4-6 yrs.		X		X			X	
11-12 yrs.								
Total	3	5	4	4	4	annually	2	1

Table 3:
Recommended Childhood and Adolescent Vaccination Schedule 2005[3]

In the late 1700s, each year one million people died in Europe alone from a devastating disease called smallpox, especially children. Many who were not killed lived with severe effects from the disease, including blindness and deformities. During this time an English physician by the name of Edward Jenner made a remarkable observation. Jenner recognized that milkmaids who worked with cows affected with a similar disease called cowpox did not become infected with smallpox. Jenner carried out a very important experiment. He took fluid from the pustule of a woman infected with cowpox and injected it into a healthy child that had never contracted smallpox or cowpox. Several weeks later he injected fluid from a smallpox pustule into the child, and the child remained healthy. Jenner's experiment laid the foundation for the development of modern vaccines. Millions no longer suffer from the effects of severe diseases such as smallpox. Since Jenner's discovery, many vaccines have been developed and licensed for use to prevent many serious, even fatal diseases. Table 3 provides a list of licensed vaccines in use at the time of this writing. However, this is an area that will be continuously updated.

Types of vaccines

You may be interested in learning about the different types of vaccines currently in use. Below is a list that briefly explains the differences between each type.

- *Inactivated* (killed) vaccines contain dead germs; they cannot multiply and spread in our bodies. Our bodies are able to recognize that they are foreign and mount a specific immune response to them.
- *Live attenuated* vaccines contain germs that have been altered or weakened in some way. They are able to get into the body and trigger an immune response, but are unable to multiply well enough to cause a severe infection. Sometimes they can cause minor symptoms of the disease, but they are usually not as severe as infection with the living germs.
- *Subunit* vaccines are nonliving and contain only a part of the germ (antigen), which triggers an immune response.
- *Toxoid* vaccines contain a chemical that will stimulate the body's immune system to act against those chemicals (toxins) when they are secreted from bacteria.
- *Recombinant* vaccines are produced in germs such as bacteria. Scientists have learned how to use these germs to produce proteins that are very similar to the actual proteins of germs that cause disease.
- *Multivalent* vaccines are "cocktails," or mixtures, containing vaccines for several different types of germs. They may include a combination of the different types described above. The measles, mumps, and rubella, or MMR, vaccine is an example.

It is important to include a small disclaimer here: there are no vaccines that are completely, 100 percent safe or effective. Each person's immune system may react differently, and there is no way to predict how each person will react. Some people do not respond to vaccination at all, while others may develop allergic reactions. Still others may experience the side effects that were mentioned previously. It all depends on each person's reaction.

The controversy

Although the number of cases is considerably low, there have been some reports of serious illness and even death associated with vaccine use. For this reason the Vaccine Injury Compensation Act was passed in 1986. It became funded in 1988. This fund awards cash benefits to families that have children who have suffered from severe injury such as brain damage or death due to vaccination.

A recent area of concern for vaccines has been a potential link to autism. The Department of Education reports that from school years 1991–1992 to 2001–2002 the number of children in the United States diagnosed with autism increased from 5,415 to 118,602.[4] The increase for cases of autism was greater than that for all other disabilities in general. Some groups have suggested that the MMR (mumps, measles, and rubella) vaccine and thimerosal, a mercury-based preservative, are linked to autism. These claims have not been supported by definitive experimental data. Also, there have been no harmful effects reported for thimerosal used at the doses recommended for vaccines.

Several groups have investigated the link between the MMR vaccine and autism and have reported that there is none. In one study, researchers in London analyzed the trends of autism in the population after use of the MMR vaccine. They concluded that there is no causal association between the MMR vaccine and autism.[5] In a study in Denmark, more than seven hundred children were identified who had either autism or autistic-spectrum disorders. The investigators compared the vaccinated and unvaccinated groups of children with the disorders and concluded that the evidence is against the MMR vaccine causing autism.[6] A recent study conducted at the University of London examined 2,407 people born between 1959 and 1993 to determine if there was increased risk of autism after exposure to measles virus or several different types of MMR vaccines. They concluded that there was no increased risk of autism after exposure to measles virus and measles vaccines.[7]

Since 1999 the number of thimerosal-based vaccines has been decreased. To date there is no clear explanation for the increase in cases of autism, nor is there a clear understanding as to what causes the condition.

What is clear is that many of the infectious diseases that were once debilitating or even fatal are now preventable because of vaccines. They are most effective when they are given according to the recommended schedule and given to most of the people in a given community. They are not *perfect*; nothing is perfect. Cases of mild to severe side effects have been reported, and some vaccines have been recalled for this reason. One important thing to remember is that researchers are continuing to conduct studies to improve vaccines and ensure their safety and efficacy. The FDA and CDC continue to monitor the safety and efficacy of vaccines that are currently on the market. As a parent, it is important to read the literature provided by the physician and ask questions if there is something that you are unsure of when having your children immunized.

Why should you feel safe about vaccines that are in use today?

There should be some comfort in knowing that it is not easy to get a vaccine approved for widespread use. The FDA requires that vaccines be tested extensively to ensure safety before licensure for general use. It may take from ten to fifty years from the time a vaccine is discovered until the time it is approved. Prior to testing in humans, a vaccine must first be tested in laboratory animals such as mice and rabbits. It must then be approved for clinical trials in humans through an extensive application process. If approved for licensure and placed on the market, the FDA continues to monitor its safety. As the number of vaccinated people increases, research studies are conducted involving larger numbers to measure its efficacy and safety. Finally, the Vaccine Adverse Events Reporting System (VAERS) is used by the FDA and CDC to gather information about licensed vaccines. This system is designed so that doctors, patients, and others may report any unusual reactions, symptoms, or complications associated with a vaccine. The FDA views weekly VAERS reports for unusual reports about vaccines that are currently in use.

GERM TIP #8:
The types of vaccines licensed to prevent infectious diseases caused by germs are:
- Inactivated or killed vaccines
- Live attenuated vaccines
- Subunit vaccines
- Toxoid vaccines
- Recombinant vaccines

WHAT ARE TREATMENTS?

Treatments are remedies developed and prescribed to provide temporary relief for the symptoms associated with infection. A treatment differs from prevention in that it is designed to target the symptoms of the disease. Treatments do not prevent diseases from occurring. Physicians recommend treatments for illnesses, and often there are no guarantees. Naturally we should seek a professional to treat our illnesses, but spiritually, we should first seek the Lord. Do not by any means place all of your faith in physicians. Physicians are human, after all, and are capable of error just like you and me. The Bible gives us an example of a king named Asa who had a disease and chose to put all of his faith in a physician *instead* of the Lord.

> And, behold, the acts of Asa, first and last, lo, they are written in the book of the kings of Judah and Israel. And Asa in the thirty and ninth year of his reign was diseased in his feet, until his disease was exceeding great: yet in his disease he sought not to the LORD, but to the physicians. And Asa slept with his fathers, and died in the one and fortieth year of his reign.
> —2 CHRONICLES 16:11–13

Cold medicine, flu medicine, cold and flu medicine, sinus medicine, sinus and cold medicine—today you can walk into any drugstore or supermarket and find drugs to treat just about any ailment imaginable. There was a time when many of the medicines that are sold over the counter today required a prescription from a physician. It required more time and perhaps more money to get the medicine, but you felt confident that you had the right treatment for the condition. Today there is such a large selection to choose from that it can be somewhat confusing. People spend a great deal of time attempting to select the correct medicine. With the advancements in drug research and the pharmaceutical drug industry, there are many treatments available for the common illnesses caused by germs. This section was written to help you to make educated choices when buying over-the-counter drugs. It is also strongly recommended that you speak with a pharmacist when you have questions and when selecting drugs for symptoms associated with infectious diseases.

Antihistamines and decongestives

Antihistamines are drugs that we take to provide temporary relief from such symptoms as sneezing, runny nose, and watery eyes. They work specifically to block the actions of histamines, compounds in our bodies that work as part of the immune system and are involved in inflammation. Generally, they are used for allergies, but people often use them for cold and flu-like symptoms. An example of an antihistamine is chlorpheniramine maleate, found in cold medicines such as Triaminic or Robitussin.

Decongestives work specifically to break down mucus and clear our nasal passages, providing us with the ability to breathe more easily. An example of a nasal decongestant is pseudoephedrine HCl, which is also an active ingredient of cold medicines. Previously, I mentioned that many of these symptoms are caused by our immune system and help us to clear the infection. Therefore, taking antihistamines and decongestives actually impede the immune system and may cause it to take longer to clear the actual infection. Since the symptoms associated with infection are uncomfortable, most people prefer to take drugs and have temporary relief from the symptoms, even if it means that it may take a little longer to clear the infection.

Acetaminophen and ibuprofen

In addition to the drugs described previously, other drugs are used in combination with them or in addition to them. Acetaminophen is a fever reducer and a mild pain reliever. Fever is one of the first signs of infection, and, if excessive, it can cause severe damage to cells of the nervous system or even death. But fever is also part of the physiological defenses of the immune system. Often many medicines include acetaminophen as a fever reducer in addition to the other active ingredients.

Ibuprofen is used to relieve the swelling of inflammation (anti-inflammatory). It may also be used as a fever reducer and mild pain reliever. Tylenol is an example of a brand that contains acetaminophen, while Motrin is an example of a brand that contains ibuprofen.

Antibiotics and antifungals

It's 3:00 a.m., and your child walks into your bedroom to awaken you from a restful slumber. Half groggy, you stumble out of bed to realize that he is burning up with fever. The thermometer reading is 102° F. The same day, you rush your child to the pediatrician's office so that your child is the first patient seen. He shows all the symptoms of a "bug": coughing, fever, listlessness, and runny nose. You're *sure* the doctor will give him an antibiotic. After waiting for an hour and then consulting with the doctor for a brief ten minutes, the doctor says, "It's just a virus. There's nothing that I can give him. We'll just have to let it run its course." Twenty dollars and five hours later, you're sent home empty-handed.

But the truth is the pediatrician is right. If you or your child have a cold or the flu, antibiotics won't work. Illnesses such as colds, flu, chest colds, and sore throats (except for strep throat) are caused by *viruses,* not *bacteria*, which is why prescribing an antibiotic is more harmful than good.

Antibiotics are compounds that kill or inhibit the growth of bacteria. *Antibiotics do not work for infections caused by viruses or other germs.* Depending on the nature of the infection, they may be used in the form of an oral drug (pill or liquid), topical ointment, or in severe cases, as in the case of Jenna, an injection. They act to kill bacteria in one of three ways: destroying the bacterial cell wall, preventing bacteria from making proteins, or preventing the bacteria from making DNA. You may recall that bacteria come in a variety of forms, shapes, and types. Antibiotics are grouped according to how they act to destroy the bacteria and by the types of bacteria that they target. For example, penicillin and ampicillin are antibiotics that affect the bacterial cell wall. Other examples are tetracycline, which prevents bacteria from making proteins, and ciprofloxacin, which stops the bacteria from making DNA. Antibiotics are prescribed by physicians for a variety of illnesses, and, if taken properly, they are very effective.

Antifungals are drugs that are used to treat fungal infections. Like antibiotics, they may be taken orally or topically. Antifungals act to destroy fungi in the same manner that antibiotics kill bacteria; they are specific for some component of the fungi's makeup or target the production of a necessary compound for the fungi. For example, allylamines are antifungals that inhibit the production of sterols, substances needed for the fungi to survive. There are also drugs prescribed that specifically target sugars necessary for survival of fungi. Antifungals are typically very effective when diligence is applied. Depending on the type of infection, they may be prescribed for use over long periods of time.

Antiviral and parasitic treatments

Antiviral drugs act differently than antibiotics and antifungals. Many antiviral drugs target the proteins (enzymes) that the virus uses to copy itself. These drugs, called analogues, work to prevent the virus from multiplying and infecting other cells. Acyclovir, an antiviral used to treat herpes, is an analogue that targets the protein that copies the viral genetic material. Another example is ritonavir, an antiviral used to treat HIV infections. It targets the protein that is used to process the viral proteins.

Treatments for infections caused by parasites vary and cannot be placed into one specific group. This is because parasites vary greatly in types and sizes. Also, parasites may infect a variety of tissue types and cause varying degrees of damage. The recommended treatment is based on the type of parasite and the infected tissues. Pain relievers are usually prescribed to provide temporary relief for the pain and symptoms associated with many of the infections caused by parasites. It is very important to understand and follow the instructions for the treatments described. The Bible tells us to seek wisdom and under-standing and that following instructions keep us safe and in good health. (See Proverbs 4.)

> Take fast hold of instruction; let her not go: keep
> her; for she is thy life.... For they are life unto
> those that find them, and health to all their flesh.
> —PROVERBS 4:13, 22

GERM TIP #9

The common treatments for infections by germs are:
- Antihistamines and decongestives—allergies, cold and flu-like symptoms
- Acetaminophen and ibuprofen—fever reducers and mild pain relievers
- Antibiotics and antifungals—bacterial and fungal infections
- Antivirals and antiparasitic drugs—viral and parasitic infections

WHAT ARE THE SIDE EFFECTS?

It is important to mention that not all germs cause infection in their hosts. There are actually some germs that reside in—and on—our bodies that are not harmful. Actually they are quite help-ful in fighting off infection from other germs that are in competi-tion for the same space in or on our bodies. We call these germs a part of our *normal flora*, and we maintain a mutually beneficial (symbiotic) relationship with them. They live in or on us and are benefited by the conditions of our bodies, while we benefit by their protection from harmful germs.

One possible side effect of taking prescribed medications such as antibiotics is that they may not only kill the harmful bacteria, but may also kill the helpful bacteria. As a result the harmful germs are then able to cause infection because they are no longer in competi-tion with the helpful germs for the space. As a matter of fact, some germs that are not normally infectious are able to cause infection simply because they can. These germs are called opportunists (opportunistic pathogens); they cause infection when they have the opportunity.

A second side effect of some medications is drowsiness. Many of the drugs recommended for relief of cold and flu-like symptoms include substances that cause drowsiness. Be sure to read labels carefully to ensure that you are aware of the side effects. It is not recommended that you drive or perform any activities that require you to be alert. If you are unsure, ask a pharmacist for help. Also, doctors do not always inform us of the possible opportunistic infections that may occur as a result of taking prescribed medications. Sometimes people don't ask questions because they feel intimidated by the amount of knowledge the doctor has on the subject or because they have fear that they will not understand if they ask. It is very important to ask questions. These situations are opportunities to pray for God to provide you with confidence and understanding. Be sure to use the right approach; patiently and politely ask questions until you have a complete understanding. It is all part of taking care of your temple.

Chapter 14

TAKING CARE OF THE TEMPLE

Just as it is with anything else that needs preventative mainte-
nance, we must take care of our bodies if we want them to work
well. The Bible is very clear about the fact that our bodies are temples for God. We should take care of them!

> What? know ye not that your body is the temple of
> the Holy Ghost which is in you, which ye have of
> God, and ye are not your own? For ye are bought
> with a price: therefore glorify God in your body,
> and in your spirit, which are God's.
>   —1 Corinthians 6:19–20

There are things that we can do naturally to help our bodies
maintain healthiness, thus decreasing our chances of illnesses and
infections. But it is also important to maintain a healthy spiritual
life by applying the practices described in the previous chapters.
The Bible describes the rewards of applying discipline in our lives.

> He openeth also their ear to discipline, and com-
> mandeth that they return from iniquity. If they
> obey and serve him, they shall spend their days in
> prosperity, and their years in pleasures.
>   —Job 36:10–11

It requires discipline and diligence, but it is well worth the
reward. In this chapter we will cover the physical aspects of preventing diseases. The next chapter will cover the spiritual aspect of
prevention in more detail.

WASH YOUR HANDS

One of the best ways to prevent infectious diseases has been mentioned in almost every chapter of this book. It is so simple that

many people don't consider the health benefits. It is hand washing. Hand washing is effective and takes very little time. Below is CDC's recommendation for effective hand washing.[1]

- First, wet your hands and apply liquid or clean bar soap. Place the bar soap on a rack and allow it to drain.
- Next rub your hands together vigorously and scrub all surfaces, including between your fingers and under your fingernails.
- Continue for 10–15 seconds or about the length of a short tune. The soap combined with the scrubbing action helps dislodge and remove germs.
- Rinse well, and dry your hands.

You should wash your hands:

- Before, during, and after you prepare food
- Before you eat
- After you use the bathroom
- After changing a diaper
- After handling animals or animal waste
- When your hands are dirty
- Frequently when caring for a sick person

Washing your hands and encouraging your loved ones to wash their hands is probably the best thing that you can do to help them prevent infectious diseases. Parents should try to encourage their children to wash their hands as often as possible. It is never too late to begin healthy habits, and hand washing is one of the best.

KEEPING YOUR ENVIRONMENT "GERM FREE"

Part of taking care of yourself is taking care of your environment. It is important to take care of areas where you spend your time—workplace, home, or automobile. I would like to offer some suggestions that may help. First, remember that there is a difference between *cleaning* and *disinfecting*. Cleaning is the removal of dirt, while disinfecting is killing germs. There is a difference, but I am sure you would like to do both in your environment.

What can I do to keep my environment "germ free"?

To clean your environment, use detergents (soap). These products are very effective at removing dirt and may also be effective at killing some, but not all, germs.

To disinfect your environment, use bleach-based products. An inexpensive and effective way to kill germs in your environment is to use 10 percent bleach as a disinfectant. Ten percent bleach is effective at killing almost all germs. You may purchase a squirt bottle and make a disinfectant using one part bleach to nine parts water. *Note*: The bleach solution will lose its effectiveness after a while, so make a fresh disinfectant batch routinely, at least once a week. Also, be careful around other household members and pets.

Sterilization is another method of killing germs. If you have a dishwasher, use it. Dishwashers have heating coils so the water in a dishwasher gets much hotter than the water from your kitchen sink. Remember, many germs don't like high temperatures. A dishwasher is about the best thing that you can do to sterilize dishes and utensils in your home. Most dishwashers today have a cycle for sanitizing or sterilizing dishes. *Note*: Please use water conservatively. It is wasteful to run a dishwasher that is less than half full.

How do I properly disinfect areas?

First, clean surfaces with soap using a sponge. Sponges dry quickly and completely and are less likely to house germs in comparison to cloths. Why? They do not retain moisture, but do retain soap scum and many germs don't like that. Second, spray with disinfectant and wipe dry with a paper towel.

When should I clean and disinfect?

Frequently clean and disinfect surfaces that are likely to have lots of germs. For example, you may choose to spray surfaces in your kitchen and bathroom daily. This takes very little time using a squirt bottle and paper towels.

EATING RIGHT

As described previously, some of the germs that cause disease in our bodies are transmitted in foods. It is therefore important that we apply preventive methods to decrease the chances of infection by controlling *how* we eat. Below is a list of practical methods that can decrease the risk of infectious disease contracted from foods.

- Always wash your hands before eating.
- Disinfect surfaces used to prepare foods. (Use bleach-based products.)
- Clean all cooking and eating utensils with detergents.
- Eat in clean environments.
- Cook foods completely, especially meats.

The Bible is very clear about how to prepare the food preparation areas, take care of utensils, and prepare food before eating. This scripture gives specific instructions on the Jewish custom of hand washing before eating.

> And when they come from the market, except they wash, they eat not. And many other things there be, which they have received to hold, as the washing of cups, and pots, brasen vessels, and of tables.
>
> —MARK 7:4

Another scripture gives specific instruction about not eating blood.

> Moreover ye shall eat no manner of blood, whether it be of fowl or of beast, in any of your dwellings.
> —LEVITICUS 7:26

Food products with blood are not healthy because blood caries nutrients and waste through an organism. When we eat blood we are endangering our own lives. We can also increase our chances of healthiness and decrease our chances of infection by controlling what we eat.

A major factor in good health is nutrition. Nutritional experts describe specific foods that are not good for us to eat. Fats provide our bodies with energy and provide vitamins A, D, E, K, and carotenoids. However, these vitamins are only obtained from foods with unsaturated fats. Unsaturated fats are oils and may be obtained from foods such as vegetables, fish, and nuts. This is why it is highly recommended that we cook our foods in vegetable oils. These are the good fats. Saturated fats do not help absorb vitamins and tend to raise blood cholesterol. High blood cholesterol levels may lead to complications, including coronary heart disease. You can decrease your intake of saturated fats by doing the following:

- Use low-fat or no-fat dairy products such as cheese, cream, butter, and milk.
- Avoid fatty meats and remove the skin from poultry before cooking.
- Avoid eating red meat with marbled fat and organ meats.
- Avoid margarine and shortening whenever possible.

The Word of God is very specific about what we should and should not eat.

> Speak unto the children of Israel, saying, Ye shall eat no manner of fat, of ox, or of sheep, or of goat. ... And the swine, though he divide the hoof, and be clovenfooted, yet he cheweth not the cud; he is unclean to you. Of their flesh shall ye not eat, and their carcase shall ye not touch; they are unclean to you.
>
> —LEVITICUS 7:23; 11:7–8

We help to determine the ability of our bodies to work for us and fight off diseases partly by what we put into them. If we do not supply them with the right nutrition, we cannot expect them to do a good job. The reward for obedience and discipline in this area is good health.

EAT TO LIVE

Part of maintaining good health is to decrease our food intake especially if we are overweight. Being overweight increases blood pressure in people who have high blood pressure (hypertension). Moreover, there is mounting evidence that fat stored within the abdomen around the vital organs leads to the increased production of inflammatory cytokines that promote atherosclerosis and sap the strength of the immune system to defend against the enemy (*germs* and abnormal cancer cells). The 2PD Omer Approach is one way to decrease your food intake if you are overweight (chapter ten). This approach is proven to work and helps people to develop discipline in other areas of their lives. Curbing your appetite and desire to overeat is important so that you eat when you are hungry, not when you are emotional. We do not live on food alone, but on every word that comes from God. (See Deuteronomy 8:3.) This is the same scripture that our Lord Jesus Christ spoke when the devil tempted Him during His forty-day fast in the desert. (See Matthew 4:4.)

Those who have specific medical conditions such as hypertension or diabetes should also follow their physician's dietary advice restricting sodium and sugar, respectively. These restrictions are easily incorporated into reductions in overall food intake. Indeed, some people find that it is easier to eat less when the food is bland because of less salt and sugar.

Therefore, it is very important that we have an understanding of what is good.

> Understanding is a wellspring of life unto him that
> hath it: but the instruction of fools is folly.
> —PROVERBS 16:22

Eating the right amount and kinds of foods increases our chances of maintaining good health, which can help us to fight infection.

SUGGESTIONS FOR EATING RIGHT

Here is a suggested list of things you can do to make sure you eat the right foods.

- Eat foods from each of the food groups: fruits and vegetables, cereal and grains, dairy products, and proteins.
- Limit your intake of foods that are high in saturated fats such as fatty meats and whole-fat dairy products such as cheese and butter.

- Limit your food intake, especially if you are over-weight. The 2PD Omer Approach is one simple way.
- Avoid snacking between meals. Try drinking water and meditating on Scripture instead.
- Work hard to monitor how much you are eating.

RESTING

Most of us live hectic, stressful lives. People who live under stressful conditions appear to be more susceptible to infections than people living under less stressful conditions. That is why getting the proper rest is an important part of caring for our bodies. We cannot expect our bodies to work hard to defend us from infectious diseases if we do not take care of them. We must set aside time to rest our bodies. The Word of God tells us that we are not to work continuously, but rather we must set aside specific time for rest.

> Six days thou shalt do thy work, and on the seventh day thou shalt rest: that thine ox and thine ass may rest, and the son of thy handmaid, and the stranger, may be refreshed.
>
> —Exodus 23:12

A refreshed body is more equipped to work for us.

EXERCISING

For some people getting started is so difficult, but once they do start exercising, they immediately begin to reap the benefits, and it motivates them to continue. According to the U.S. Public Health Service, physical fitness and exercise is one of the fifteen areas of greatest importance for improving the health of the public.[2]

It doesn't have to be something that you dread doing. If you have not incorporated exercise into your life, try to find some fun way to do so. Some examples of exercises that could be incorporated into busy schedules are walking, swimming, jogging, cycling, and lifting weights. Each person is different and must develop a program that works best for him or her, but everyone can benefit from regular exercise. Exercising is a natural way to take care of the body.

The first step in incorporating an exercise plan into your life is to make the commitment. It must be something that you have decided to do because you need to and something that you plan to stick with. It will require time, effort, and patience to be successful. If you are a beginner, do not try to do too much too soon. Also, be prepared for it to take some time before you see the results. If you are willing to make the commitment and practice patience, you will see that it is far worth the reward.

The Bible is very clear about the fact that our bodies are temples for God. We should take care of them!

> What? know ye not that your body is the temple of the Holy Ghost which is in you, which ye have of God, and ye are not your own? For ye are bought with a price: therefore glorify God in your body, and in your spirit, which are God's.
> —1 Corinthians 6:19–20

Help to maintain good health and decrease the risk of infection with germs by:
- Washing your hands
- Taking care of your environment
- Eating right
- Resting
- Exercising

GERM TIP #10

To be healthy includes being free of disease, injury, and stress. Our overall health depends greatly on the decisions we make. God grants each of us the option to choose. Maintaining a healthy lifestyle depends greatly on the choices we make. We can choose to eat right, rest, exercise, and decrease the stress in our lives. Practicing healthy behaviors contributes to our well-being and can greatly reduce the risk of infections and illness. In a similar manner, practicing spiritual concepts contributes to a healthy attitude.

Chapter 15

PRAYER AND A GOOD ATTITUDE

Hearing, reading, and meditating on the Word of God, as well as assembling in fellowship, are all practices that will help in our prayer life. They are practices that we should develop. It requires both dedication and discipline. In doing so, we develop our relationship with God by learning about Him through His Word. We become familiar with His will for our lives. This enables us to pray and ask for His will in our lives. We may pray for good health for ourselves and loved ones in faith believing that we will receive what we ask. The Bible tells us in Mark 11:24 that when praying, we should ask for the desires of our hearts in faith, believing that we will receive what we ask for. Therefore we should continuously pray for the things we want in our lives and the lives of our loved ones that are aligned with the Word of God.

> Pray without ceasing.
>
> —1 THESSALONIANS 5:17

PRAYER

I can recall my spiritual father teaching that prayer is asking God to do what is promised in His Word. For that to happen we must become familiar with His Word. The only way to truly learn the Word of God and to have faith in it is to hear it, read it, meditate on it, and fellowship with other believers.

Hear it

> So then faith cometh by hearing, and hearing by the word of God.
>
> —ROMANS 10:17

To hear the Word of God to build up faith as described in the Bible means that we must be around people that speak the Word of God, or we must receive it from other sources. An example is receiving it through a message at a local church. Listening to audiotapes, CDs, videotapes or DVDs, and television broadcasts are other examples. It is important, too, that we are selective about what we spend time listening to and that it is in agreement with the Bible.

Read it

> Till I come, give attendance to reading, to exhortation, to doctrine.
>
> —1 TIMOTHY 4:13

Reading the Bible is a practice that every Christian should develop. There is no better way to become acquainted with the Word of God than to read it. When I was younger, it was difficult for me to understand the Bible. I was not quite sure where to begin reading. I was sure that I shouldn't use the approach that I used for other books—start at the beginning and continue reading until the end. Honestly, I tried this approach rather unsuccessfully. What I learned later is that we should be led as to what to read in the Bible. Well, how are we led? One way is to become connected with a local church. If you are not a member of a church already, you may want to begin visiting churches until you find the one that is right for you. Your pastor or church leader will guide you in the direction that you should go. They may often refer to scriptures that you can later take the time and read carefully for yourself. When you are in the right place you will know because the message will agree with your spirit. Another approach is to purchase a concordance. A concordance is a helpful reference tool when you are interested in reading about a particular topic and are not sure where to find it in the Bible.

Meditate on it

> My hands also will I lift up unto thy commandments, which I have loved; and I will meditate in thy statutes.
>
> —PSALM 119:48

To *meditate* means "to ponder" or reflect on something. Therefore to meditate on the Word of God means to take time and think about it. Let it sink in, if you will. One approach is to read a scripture several times, then stop and think about it. Begin to dissect the scripture so that you completely understand it. Sometimes it requires using other references such as a different translation to be sure you have complete understanding of the scripture. Reciting the scriptures aloud is also a helpful approach.

And fellowship

> And let us consider one another to provoke unto love and to good works: Not forsaking the assembling of ourselves together, as the manner of some is; but exhorting one another: and so much the more, as ye see the day approaching.
>
> —HEBREWS 10:24–25

Finally, we are not to forsake the assembling of ourselves. This means to come together in groups to fellowship. One interpretation of this scripture is that we should have regular church attendance or home groups for fellowship. This is a way to receive instruction on how we should operate in our daily lives. We should also spend time with other believers to help each other. You also learn from other believers and are able to build meaningful and loving relationships.

A GOOD ATTITUDE

We usually say what we are thinking. Usually what comes out of our mouths is what is on our minds. There is, therefore, great power in what we say, if we say what we are thinking. The Bible tells us that we are what we think in our hearts. (See Proverbs 23:7.) It also tells us in Genesis 11 of the possible power of the mind and imagination of man from the story of the tower of Babel. The Bible tells us that at this time all of the men on earth spoke one language. Those who settled in the east began to work together to accomplish many great things. Together they were able to make brick and build a great city. The people began to feel powerful because of what they had accomplished, and they set out to build a great tower that would reach to heaven. The Lord knew that the people were working together and believed in their hearts that they were able to do what they imagined. The Bible tells us that God confounded their language so that they could no longer communicate and work together. The people eventually left the city and scattered. The point is that we are capable of great things through our imagination—what we *think*. Much of what we think and believe we are capable of accomplishing in our lives. This is why what we say is very important, because it is what we think.

It occurred to me that many people may not feel well because they don't think good thoughts, and, therefore, they say that they do not feel well. In other words, they do not have a healthy attitude. Of course, this does not mean that when people get sick it is their fault, nor does it mean that people may simply say that they are healthy and become healthy. However, our attitudes may greatly contribute to how we feel. We must control what we think and say and be careful of what comes out of our mouths. Instead of saying things such as "I don't feel very well," say "I feel great" or "I am healthy." Rather than speaking negatively, we should speak positively and of good health for ourselves and loved ones.

> Hear; for I will speak of excellent things; and the
> opening of my lips shall be right things.
> —PROVERBS 8:6

Since what we say is what is on our minds, it is important to fill our minds with the right material. Instead of filling our minds with negative, depressing, and hopeless ideas and images, we should try to fill our minds with positive, uplifting, and hopeful ideas and images. If this is what we fill our minds with, then this is what will come out of our mouths. Studying the Bible builds faith. In doing so, we can develop a mental picture, or "vision," of good health for ourselves and our families. We will then begin to speak these things. Develop a vision of healthiness for your life and have faith in it. Just as you plan for other things in your life, you should also plan to have good health.

NOTES

INTRODUCTION

1. U.S. Department of Health and Human Services, Centers for Disease Control and Prevention, "Summary of Health Statistics for U.S. Children: National Health Interview Survey, 2002," Vital and Health Statistics 10(221): 24–25 (2004), http://www.cdc.gov/nchs/data/series/sr_10/sr10_221.pdf (accessed May 15 2004).

2. Centers for Disease Control and Prevention, "Stop the Spread of Germs," http://www.cdc.gov/germstopper/home_work_school.htm (accessed March 15, 2004).

3. Ibid.

CHAPTER 1: GERMS: WHAT THEY ARE

1. *Microbeworld,* "Viruses—and Some Virus-like Agents," http://www.microbeworld.org/htm/aboutmicro/microbes/types/virus.htm (accessed May 4, 2005).

2. J. Deacon, "The Microbial World: Bacterial Colonies, Gram Reaction, and Cell Shapes," Institute of Cell and Molecular Biology, The University of Edinburgh, http://helios.bto.ed.ac.uk/bto/microbes/shape.htm (accessed December 2, 2004).

3. Department of Parasitology, Faculty of Medicine, Chiang Mai University, Thailand, http://www.medicine.cmu.ac.th/dept/parasite/image.htm (accessed November 12, 2004).

4. Ibid.

CHAPTER 3: GERMS IN THE MEDIA

1. Centers for Disease Control and Prevention, "Questions and Answers About Anthrax," http://bt.cdc.gov/agent/anthrax/faq/ (accessed May 31, 2005).

2. U.S. Department of Health and Human Services, Centers for Disease Control and Prevention. "Bovine Spongiform Encephalopathy in a Dairy Cow—Washington State, 2003," *Morbidity and Mortality Weekly Report* 52(53): 1280–1285 (January 9, 2004), http://www.cdc.gov/mmwr/preview/mmwrhtml/mm5253a2.htm (accessed November 17, 2004).

3. Centers for Disease Control and Prevention, "Severe Acute Respiratory Syndrome (SARS)," http://www.cdc.gov/ncidod/sars/factsheet.htm (accessed November 17, 2004).

4. Centers for Disease Control and Prevention, "2004 West Nile Virus Activity in the United States," http://www.cdc.gov/ncidod/dvbid/westnile/surv&controlCaseCount04_detailed.htm (accessed May 1, 2005).

5. Centers for Disease Control and Prevention, "West Nile Virus: What You Need To Know," http://www.cdc.gov/ncidod/dvbid/westnile/wnv_factsheet.htm (accessed November 17, 2005).

CHAPTER 4: COLDS AND FLU

1. S. Cohen, et. al., "Psychological Stress and Susceptibility to the Common Cold," *New England Journal of Medicine* 325(9) (August 1991): 606–612.

2. Centers for Disease Control and Prevention, "Key Facts About the Flu: How to Prevent the Flu and What to Do If You Get Sick," http://www.cdc.gov/flu/keyfacts.htm (accessed March 15, 2005).

3. Centers for Disease Control and Prevention, "All Children 6 to 23 Months Old Should Get Flu Shot," http://www.cdc.gov/flu/protect/infants.htm (accessed May 20, 2004).

4. E. P. Gurfinkel, et. al., "Two-Year Follow-Up of the Flu Vaccination Acute Coronary Syndromes (FLUVACS) Registry," *Tex Heart Inst J.* 31(1) (2004): 28–32.

CHAPTER 5: PNEUMONIA

1. Centers for Disease Control and Prevention, "Drug-resistant *Streptococcus pneumoniae* Disease," http://www.cdc.gov/ncidod/dbmd/diseaseinfo/drugresisstreppneum_t.htm (accessed March 15, 2004).

2. Centers for Disease Control and Prevention, "Infectious Disease Information, Pneumonia," http://www.cdc.gov/ncidod/diseases/submenus/sub_pneumonia.htm (accessed March 15, 2004).

CHAPTER 6: EAR AND THROAT INFECTIONS

1. Centers for Disease Control and Prevention, "Group A Streptococcal (GAS) Disease," http://www.cdc.gov/ncidod/dbmd/diseaseinfo/groupastreptococcal_g.htm (accessed May 1, 2005).

2. Centers for Disease Control and Prevention, "Epstein-Barr Virus and Infectious Mononucleosis," http://www.cdc.gov/ncidod/diseases/ebv.htm (accessed March 14, 2004).

3. Ibid.

CHAPTER 7: DIARRHEA

1. R. L. Fankhauser, et. al., "Epidemiologic and Molecular Trends of 'Norwalk-like Viruses' Associated With Outbreaks of Gastroenteritis in the United States," *Journal of Infectious Diseases* 186(1) (July 2002): 1–7.

2. Centers for Disease Control and Prevention, "Chronic Diarrhea," Parasitic Disease Information, http://www.cdc.gov/ncidod/dpd/parasites/diarrhea/factsht_chronic_diarrhea.htm (accessed March 19, 2004).

CHAPTER 8: SEXUALLY TRANSMITTED DISEASES

1. Centers for Disease Control and Prevention, "STD Surveillance 2003 National Profile, Chlamydia," http://www.cdc.gov/std/stats/chlamydia.htm (accessed May 5, 2005).

2. Centers for Disease Control and Prevention, "STD Surveillance 2003 Special Focus Profiles, Adolescents and Young Adults," http://www.cdc.gov/std/stats/adol.htm (accessed May 5, 2005).

3. Centers for Disease Control and Prevention, *Sexually Transmitted Disease Surveillance 2003 Supplement, Syphilis Surveillance Report* (Atlanta, GA: U.S. Department of Health and Human Services, Centers for Disease Control and Prevention, December 2004).

4. Centers for Disease Control and Prevention, "Male Latex Condoms and Sexually Transmitted Disease," http://www.cdc.gov/nchstp/od/latex.htm (accessed May 8, 2004).

CHAPTER 10: CANCER

1. "Cancer Statistics 2005," American Cancer Society, http://www.cancer.org/docroot/PRO/content/PRO_/_/Cancer_Statistics_2005_Presentation.asp (accessed June 13, 2005).

2. "Detailed Guide: Cancer (General Information), Who Gets Cance?" American Cancer Society, Inc., http://www.cancer.org/docroot/CRI/content/CRI_2_4_1x_Who_gets_cancer.asp?sitearea= (accessed October 15, 2004).

3. "Detailed Guide: Cancer (General Information), What Are the Risk Factors for Cancer?" American Cancer Society, Inc., http://www.cancer.org/docroot/CRI/content/CRI_2_4_2x_What_are_the_risk_factors_for_cancer_72.asp?sitearea= (accessed October 15, 2004).

4. Ibid.

5. Centers for Disease Control and Prevention, "Viral Hepatitis B," http://www.cdc.gov/ncidod/diseases/hepatitis/b/fact.htm (accessed May 5, 2005).

6. Ibid.

7. A. B. Chung, "History Behind the 2PD-Omer Approach," http://www.heartmdphd.com/wtloss.asp (accessed January 24, 2005).

CHAPTER 11: ACQUIRED IMMUNODEFICIENCY SYNDROME (AIDS)

1. U.S. Department of Health and Human Services, National Institutes of Health, "HIV Infection and AIDS: An Overeview," http://www.niaid.nih.gov/factsheets/hivinf.htm (accessed January 30, 2005).

2. Ibid.

CHAPTER 12: DISEASES OF MAJOR ORGANS AND TISSUES

1. S. O'Connor, et. al., "Potential Infectious Etiologies of Atherosclerosis: A Mulitfactoral Perspective," *Emerging Infectious Diseases* 7(5) (September–October 2001): 780–788.

2. Ibid.

3. C. A. Gaydos, et. al., "The Role of *Chlamydia Pneumoniae* in Cardiovascular Disease," *Advances in Internal Medicine* 45 (2000): 139–173.

4. J. B. Muhlestein, et. al., "Infection With Chlamydia Pneumoniae Accelerates the Development of Atherosclerosis and Treatment With Azithromycin Prevents It in a Rabbit Model," *Circulation* 97(7) (February 1998): 633–636.

5. L. A. Campbell, et. al., "*Chlamydia pneumoniae* and Cardiovascular Disease," *Emerging Infectious Diseases* 4(4) (October–December 1998): 571–579.

6. Centers for Disease Control and Prevention, "Diabetes Public Health," http://www.cdc.gov/diabetes/statistics/prev/national/figpersons.htm (accessed November 19, 2004).

7. H. Kawashima et. al., "Enterovirus-Related Type 1 Diabetes Mellitus and Antibodies to Glutamic Acid Decarboxylase in Japan," *Journal of Infectious Diseases* 49(2) (August 2004): 147–151.

8. B. Schwartz. "Arthritis: Other, Lyme Disease," http://www.hopkins-arthritis.som.jhmi.edu/other/lyme.html (accessed May 3, 2005).

9. Ibid.

10. Centers for Disease Control and Prevention, "*Helicobacter pylori* and Peptic Ulcer Disease," http://www.cdc.gov/ulcer/ (accessed May 4, 2005).

CHAPTER 13: PREVENTION VS. TREATMENT

1. Centers for Disease Control and Prevention, "Six Common Misconceptions About Vaccines and How to Respond to Them," http://www.cdc.gov/nip/publications/6mishome.htm (accessed May 17, 2004).

2. Ibid.

3. Centers for Disease Control and Prevention, "Recommended Childhood and Adolescent Immunization Schedule, United States—2005," National Immunization Program, http://www.cdc.gov/nip/recs/child-schedule.htm (accessed April 14, 2005).

4. F. Edward Yazbak, "Autism in the United States, a Perspective," United States Department of Education, http://www.jpands.org/vol8no4/yazbak.pdf (accessed November 18, 2004).

5. B. Taylor, et. al., "Autism and Measles, Mumps, and Rubella Vaccine: No Epidemiological Evidence for a Causal Association," *Lancet* 353 (9169) (June 2000): 2026–2029.

6. K. M. Madsen, et. al., "A Population-based Study of Measles, Mumps, and Rubella Vaccination and Autism," *New England Journal of Medicine* 347(19) (November 2002): 1477–1482.

7. W. Chen, et. al., "No Evidence for Links Between Autism, MMR and Measles Virus," *Psychological Medicine* 34(3) (April 2004): 543–553.

CHAPTER 14: TAKING CARE OF THE TEMPLE

1. Centers for Disease Control and Prevention, "An Ounce of Prevention: Keeps the Germs Away," http://www.cdc.gov/ncidod/op/handwashing.htm (accessed March 15, 2004).

2. U.S. Department of Health and Human Services, Centers for Disease Control and Prevention. "Perspectives in Disease Prevention and Health Promotion Workshop on Epidemiologic and Public Health Aspects of Physical Activity and Exercise." *Morbidity and Mortality Weekly Report,* 34(13): 173–176, 181–182 (April 5, 1985). http://www.cdc.gov/mmwr/preview/mmwrhtml/00000513.htm (accessed May 17 2004).

Strang Communications, the publisher of both Charisma House and *Charisma* magazine, wants to give you 3 FREE ISSUES of our award-winning magazine.

Since its inception in 1975, *Charisma* magazine has helped thousands of Christians stay connected with what God is doing worldwide.

Within its pages you will discover in-depth reports and the latest news from a Christian perspective, biblical health tips, global events in the body of Christ, personality profiles, and so much more. Join the family of *Charisma* readers who enjoy feeding their spirit each month with miracle-filled testimonies and inspiring articles that bring clarity, provoke prayer, and demand answers.

To claim your **3 free issues** of *Charisma,* send your name and address to: Charisma 3 Free Issue Offer, 600 Rinehart Road, Lake Mary, FL 32746. Or you may call 1-800-829-3346 and ask for Offer # 93FREE. This offer is only valid in the USA.

---

www.charismamag.com